VEGAN SLOW COOKER RECIPES

Easy and Healthy Vegan Crock Pot Recipes

(Delicious and Affordable Vegan Healthy Recipes Includes Meal Plan)

Donald Hinds

Published by Sharon Lohan

© **Donald Hinds**

All Rights Reserved

Vegan Slow Cooker Recipes: Easy and Healthy Vegan Crock Pot Recipes (Delicious and Affordable Vegan Healthy Recipes Includes Meal Plan)

ISBN 978-1-990334-32-0

All rights reserved. No part of this guide may be reproduced in any form without permission in writing from the publisher except in the case of brief quotations embodied in critical articles or reviews.

Legal & Disclaimer

The information contained in this book is not designed to replace or take the place of any form of medicine or professional medical advice. The information in this book has been provided for educational and entertainment purposes only.

The information contained in this book has been compiled from sources deemed reliable, and it is accurate to the best of the Author's knowledge; however, the Author cannot guarantee its accuracy and validity and cannot be held liable for any errors or omissions. Changes are periodically made to this book. You must consult your doctor or get professional medical advice before using any of the suggested remedies, techniques, or information in this book.

Table of contents

Part 1 1

Introduction 2

Coking Tidbits 4

Meat And Dairy Alternatives 4

So, What Exactly Is Tofu? 5

Beans: Dried Or Canned? 6

Meal Plan 7

Shopping List 8

Slow Cooker Soups 12

Bisque 12

Beet Soup 14

Minestrone Soup 15

Miso Soup 17

Cauliflower Soup 18

Creamy Tomato Soup 19

Vegan Pho Soup 21

White Bean Soup 23

Split Pea Soup 25

Kidney Beans And Wild Mushroom Soup 26

Creamy Broccoli Soup 27

- Slow Cooker Main Courses 29
- Mediterranean Stuffed Peppers 29
- Pasta With Rich Sauce 31
- Indian Stuffed Pancakes 33
- Spiced Kofta In Sauce 35
- Vegan Greek Moussaka 37
- Seitan Eggplant Stew 39
- Vegetable Lasagna 41
- Burger "Steak" Balls 42
- Mushroom Tempeh Stroganoff 44
- Tofu Veggie Stew 46
- Okra Gumbo 47
- Vegan Palak Paneer 48
- Lentils Cauliflower Curry 50
- Pasta Puttanesca 52
- Lentils Veggie Rolls 53
- White Bean Quinoa Chili 55
- Lasagna Rolls 57
- Lentils Sweet Potato Stew 59
- Something Like Risotto 60
- Sweet And Sour Tofu With Quinoa 62
- Vegetables, Grains, And Beans Salads 64
- Quinoa With Grilled Pineapple 64

Delicious Ratatouille 65

Baked Beans 67

Chickpeas Salad 68

Quinoa Pilaf...70

Maple Glazed Carrots...71

Wheat Berries Bean Salad 73

Mexican Salad 74

Fresh Salad With Quinoa..76

Whole Cooked Cauliflower..77

Jacket Potatoes 79

Slow Cooker Desserts 80

Tapioca Pudding..80

Apple Crumble..81

Chocolate Fondue 82

Slow Cooked Pudding 84

Carrot Cake 85

Peached Peaches With Yogurt..87

Zebra Cake...88

Lemon Poppy Seeds Cake 90

Lazy Berry Pie...92

Lemon Dessert 94

Conclusion...95

Part 2..96

Introduction To Vegan Slow Cooking 97

Chilis, Soups, And Stews 102

Rich Mushroom And Tortellini Soup With White Sauce 102

Red Bean Noodle Soup 103

Greek Vegetable Stew With Feta Cheese 105

Spicy Vegan Chili 106

Divine Tomato And Chickpea Soup 108

Potatoes And Dumplings 110

Cheesy Potatoes Au Gratin In The Slow Cooker 110

Dumplings With Stewed Veggies 111

Savory Pies And Casseroles 113

Cheesy Tortellini Casserole With Tomato Sauce 113

Crock Pot Shepherd's Pie 114

Cheesy Slow Cooker Casserole 115

Creamy Vegetable Pie 116

Easy Crock Pot Veggie-Loaf 119

Pasta, Noodles, And Rice 122

Vegan Mushroom And Spinach Lasagna 122

Tofu Teriyaki With Steamed Rice 123

Artichoke And Tomato Fettucine 124

Tofu Peanut Surprise With Rice 125

Spicy Garbanzo Bean Curry With Brown Rice 126

Spicy Tofu-Broccoli Rice 128

Delectable Polenta And Kale Lasagna With Cheese Sauce ... 129

Mushroom Bouillon Stroganoff With Tempeh 131

Rice With Red Beans- New Orleans Style 132

Veggie-Tastic 133

Easy-Peasy Slow Cooker Burritos 133

Vegan Chinese Chow Mein 134

Grilled Tofu In Sweet And Sour Sauce With Pineapples 135

Crock Pot Vegan Pot Roast 136

Breads, Desserts, And Sweets 138

Fudgy Peanut Butter Cake 138

Crock Pot Bread Pudding 139

Heavenly Vegan Chocolate Cake 141

Lemon Blueberry Oatmeal Crock Pot Recipe 142

Apple-Cinnamon Dessert 143

Cream of Asparagus 144

Pumpkin, sweet potato and carrot soup 145

Chickpea Carrot Potato Celery Stew 146

Creamy Green Bean and Potato Soup 148

Bean Tomato Soup 149

Kale and White Bean Soup 150

Vegetable and Lentil Stew 151

Stuffed Bell Pepper in Slow Cooker 152

Bean and Pumpkin Stew 153

Chili Corn Carne...155

Potato and Olive stew 156

Hungarian Pea Stew..157

Dal Makhani...158

Carrot soup 160

Chana Masala 162

Creamy cauliflower soup with fresh chives 162

Cream of broccoli soup...164

Spicy coconut curry soup with broccoli...........................165

Zucchini Soup..166

Spinach and potato soup 167

Thick kidney bean soup 167

Mexican chili con carne..168

Kidney beans Carrot Potato Squash soup.......................169

French onion soup...171

Mushroom cream soup 172

Cream of potato with herbs and green onions 173

Thai mushroom soup..174

Fresh vegetable soup 175

Corn soup...176

Khichuri..177

Cabbage Cream Soup..178

Slow Cooker Potluck Mushrooms....................................179

Easy Slow Cooker Squash 180

Slow Cooker Tomato Sauce.. 181

Slow Cooker Jambalaya (Vegan)... 182

Breakfast 183

Slow Cooker Hash Brown Cheesy Potato Breakfast................. 183

Apple Breakfast (Easy Slow Cooker Oatmeal)........................... 184

Slow Cooker Fruit, Nuts, and Spice Oatmeal.............................. 185

Dessert 186

Slow Cooker Peach Cobbler 186

Bread Pudding in the Slow Cooker... 187

Part 1

Introduction

The truth is that you can have a happy and healthy life without eating meat, and it's easier than you might think. Studies have shown that those who eat more fruits and vegetables have a much lower risk of cancer and a lower risk of other diet-related diseases.

A Vegan diet is not as bland or dull as you might think. Most people consume more vegetables, fruits, legumes, and nuts than they think. I challenge you to try these recipes and see how many days you can go without actually eating meat.

There are many health benefits to eating a Vegan diet including:

- Helps ward of diseases, such as cancer and coronary artery disease.
- Helps maintain a lower weight.
- Longer life expectancy.
- Ease symptoms of menopause.
- More energy.
- Less toxic chemicals.
- Saves money.
- Saves animals!
- Reduces food-borne illnesses.
- Helps maintain regular bowel function.
- Helps reduce pollution.
- Enjoy a plate filled with more color.

- Easy diet to maintain.

Slow cooker meals have become a staple in many homes because they are easy and convenient. Learning to cook in a slow cooker allows you to simply throw various ingredients inside and return to a fully cooked meal hours later.

If you thought that finding meatless slow cooker recipes was challenging, these delicious recipes would change your mind.

Everyone is looking for ways to stay healthy and live longer; by eating Vegan, whether you do it every day or part of the time is a smart choice for your overall health.

So, move over classic cooking…. **Slow cooker cooking is back!** Modern cooks have discovered how to save time in the kitchen by dusting off that old slow cooker from the seventies (or buying a new one) and savoring the tantalizing aromas of healthy, home-cooked meals prepared with ease.

Slow cooking naturally lends itself to hearty stews, soups, chowders, and casseroles. Served as entrées with crusty bread and perhaps a light salad, they can make a satisfying and nutritious meal.

While Vegans appreciate the benefits of a plant-based diet, others who want to adopt a healthier eating style know that incorporating more plant-based foods is a smart way to go. Fortunately, using a slow cooker makes integrating vegetables, legumes (peas, beans), whole grains, and fruits into our daily diets, both effortless and delicious.

Most cooks know that overcooking vegetables can leave them limp, flavorless, and unappetizing. As a result, vegetable lovers have shied away from experimenting with slow cookers.

Fear no more! This cookbook is designed for everyone who wants to eat more healthfully, save time in the kitchen, and come home to a hot, nutritious meal after a long day of work or play. All that's left to figure out is what you'll do with the extra time you'll save in the kitchen!

Let's get cooking!

Coking Tidbits

Meat And Dairy Alternatives

This is a great time to be a Vegan! Those who came before us did not have the wonderful meat and dairy alternatives that are available to us today; they had to improvise their own solutions or simply do without. Fortunately, options are now flourishing in the marketplace. Dairy-free milk products run the gamut from rice milk and soya milk to coffee creamers, vegan "cheese," puddings, and frozen desserts. High-protein, healthy meat alternatives include veggie burgers and veggie dogs, burger crumbles and "ground round" loaves, roasts, links, and deli slices to suit every taste, texture, and need. I make abundant use of these nutritious foods in a wide range of my slow cooker recipes. This is because they are convenient, quick to prepare, hearty, satisfying, and generally quite low in fat.

Not all of the meat and dairy alternatives in stores are vegan (that is, completely free of animal products). If this is important to you, read product labels closely and check for animal-based ingredients such as gelatin, whey (the watery by-product of cheese making), and casein or caseinate (a milk protein that helps soy cheese "stretch" and melt.) Some manufacturers label their products as vegan, which can be extremely helpful to consumers. If a package is labeled "vegetarian," however, the product may contain dairy or egg derivatives. It is a good idea to read labels regardless, as sometimes manufacturers change their recipes or ingredients and don't indicate this clearly on the packaging.

So, What Exactly Is Tofu?

Although relatively new to the West, tofu made its first appearance in 200 BC in China. Tofu has a soft, almost cheesy texture created by curdling hot soymilk with a coagulant. A variety of agents are used to curdle the milk; these include nigari (a compound found in seawater), calcium salts (which give tofu an added calcium boost), and acidic foods such as lemon juice or vinegar. The curds are then drained and pressed into a solid block.

You can freeze and thaw tofu before using it because freezing gives tofu a chewy, spongy texture. Simply place the unopened package of tofu in the freezer until it is frozen solid; then allow it to thaw in the refrigerator. Drain it well and press it firmly between the palms of your hands to extract excess moisture before using it in recipes. Frozen tofu will turn an off-white to yellowish-brown color; this is perfectly normal and safe. If you are not using the tofu immediately after thawing; drain the water, cover the tofu with fresh water, and store it in the refrigerator. Drain the water daily and again cover the tofu with fresh water. The tofu will stay fresh for up to one week when stored this way.

Beans: Dried Or Canned?

If a recipe calls for beans, feel free to use either canned, pre-cooked, or dried beans. Canned beans are tasty, nutritious, and convenient to use. If you are watching your sodium intake, rinse canned beans well before using them, as this will remove much of the added salt.

If using dried beans, you will need to prepare them a day in advance. Dried beans must be picked over and sorted through carefully to remove any foreign objects, such as small stones or bits of twigs. Place the sorted beans in a colander and rinse them well to remove any dirt or dust. Transfer the rinsed beans to a large pot and cover them with water (the water should reach at least one or two inches above the beans) to begin the soaking process. Dried beans should be soaked for 8 to 12 hours before being cooked. After soaking, drain the beans, cover them with fresh water, and either boil them for at least 10 minutes before adding them to the slow cooker or be sure to cook them in the cooker on high the entire cook time.

Meal Plan

	Monday	Tuesday	Wednesday	Thursday	Friday	Saturday	Sunday
Entrée	Bisque	Miso Soup	Delicious Ratatouille	Split Pea Soup	Creamy Tomato Soup	Kidney Beans and Wild mushrooms Soup	Beet Soup

Main Course	Mediterranean Stuffed Peppers	Lentils Veggie Rolls	Burger "Steak" Balls	Pasta with Rich Sauce	Tofu Veggie Stew	Indian Stuffed pancakes	Pasta Puttanesca
Side Dish	...	Jacket Potatoes	Quinoa Pilaf	...	...	Baked Beans	...
Dessert	Lazy Berry Pie*	Lazy Berry Pie*	...	Chocolate Fondue	...	Tapioca pudding	Slow Cooked Pudding

*As the pie makes 12 slices, we suggest you store the remaining in the fridge and serve the following day. Chilled pie tastes amazing, with some ice cream—a true summer dessert.

Shopping List

Fruits	Avocado, 1 large

	Lemon, 1 piece
	Pomegranate, seeds, ½ cup
	Mixed berries, 5 cups
Vegetables	Corn, frozen, 2 ½ cups
	Peas, frozen, 1 cup
	Sugar peas, 1 ½ cups
	Tomatoes, beefsteak, 2
	Beets, 6
	Broccoli florets, 2 cups
	Mushrooms, button, 0.25lb
	Red cabbage, shredded, 3 cups
	Carrots, 1lb.
	Cauliflower florets, 2 cups
	Cherry tomatoes, 6
	Chili pepper, 3
	Garlic, 27 cloves
	Gold potatoes, 1lb.
	Jalapeno pepper, 1
	Leeks, 2
	Mushrooms, white, 0.5lb.
	Wild mushrooms, 1lb.
	Onion, 8
	Spring onion, 2
	Ripe tomatoes, 9lb.
	Sun-dried tomatoes, 4
	Bell peppers, any color, 4
	Red bell peppers, 3
	Yellow bell pepper, 1
	Baking potatoes, 4

	Potatoes, 2
	White potatoes, 2
	Roma tomatoes, 4
Grains	Rolled oats, 1 ½ cups
	Quinoa, cooked, 1 cup
	Quinoa, dry, 1 ¾ cups
	Wild rice, 1/3 cup
Legumes	Kidney beans, cooked, 3 ½ cups
	Brown lentils, 1 cup
	Navy beans, dried, 1lb.
Spices, Herbs &Condiments	Vanilla bean, Basil, Dried Basil, Celery flakes, Paprika powder, Bay leaf, Salt, Pepper, Thyme, Coriander, Coriander powder, Vanilla paste, Vanilla extract, Parsley, Rosemary, Cumin powder, Coconut Aminos, Balsamic vinegar, Curry powder, Garlic powder, Mustard powder, Nutmeg, Smoked paprika, Celery flakes
Oil	Coconut oil, ¾ cup
	Olive oil, 2 tablespoons
Non-dairy	Coconut cream, 1 cup
	Coconut milk, unsweetened, 1 cup
Soy products	Tofu, firm, 4oz.
	Tofu, extra-firm, 1.5lb.
Nuts and seeds	Pine nuts, 2 tablespoons
	Cashews, 1 cup
Sweeteners	Coconut sugar, ½ cup

	Maple syrup, 1/3 cup
	Molasses, 2 tablespoons
Additional	Vegan spaghetti, 8oz.
	Vegan pasta, 12oz.
	70% cacao chocolate, 4oz.
	Miso paste, 3 tablespoons
	Almond flour, ¼ cup
	Arrowroot starch, ¼ cup
	Cacao powder, 3 tablespoons
	Whole-wheat flour, ½ cup
	Tapioca pearls, ½ cup
	Black olives, 1 cup
	Palm hearts, 0.5lb
	Tomato paste, 2 tablespoons
	Vegetable stock, 19 cups
	Whole wheat flour, ½ cup
	Cornstarch, 2 tablespoons

Slow Cooker Soups

Bisque

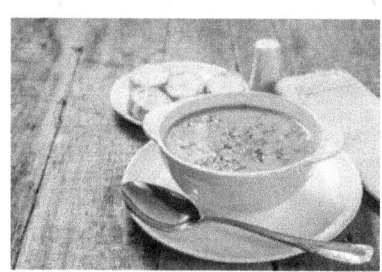

Preparation time: **10 minutes**
Cooking time: **4 hours**
Serve: 4

Ingredients:
- 0.5lb. jar palm hearts, chopped
- 4 cups vegetable stock
- 3 tablespoons coconut oil
- 2 medium leeks, washed, sliced
- 2 cloves garlic, minced
- 5 tomatoes, chopped
- 1 ½ cups frozen corn
- 1 teaspoon cayenne pepper
- ¼ cup almond flour
- ¾ cup coconut milk
- 3 tablespoons chopped parsley

Instructions:
1. heat coconut oil in a skillet.
2. Add leeks and garlic. Cook stirring for 10 minutes over medium-high heat.
3. Transfer the leeks into the slow cooker.
4. Add vegetable stock, tomatoes, corn, and cayenne pepper.
5. Set your cooker to LOW. Cook bisque for 4 hours.
6. Puree the bisque with an immersion blender.
7. In the last 30 minutes of cooking, stir in almond flour, coconut milk, and palm heart.
8. Continue to cook for 30 minutes.
9. Stir in parsley and serve warm.

Beet Soup

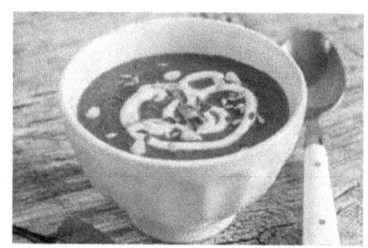

Preparation time: **10 minutes**
Cooking time: **9 hours**
Serve: 6

Ingredients:
- 6 medium beets, scrubbed
- 2 potatoes, peeled, chopped
- 1 cup carrots, peeled, cubed
- 1 red onion, sliced
- 2 tablespoons parsley, chopped
- 3 cloves garlic, minced
- 2 cups vegetable stock
- 1 cup chopped tomatoes
- 3 cups red cabbage, shredded
- Salt and pepper, to taste
- ½ cup coconut milk
- 1 tablespoon pumpkin seeds

Instructions:
1. Slice the beets and place into slow cooker.

2. Add potatoes, carrots, garlic, onion, tomatoes, and vegetable stock.
3. Season to taste with salt and pepper.
4. Cover and cook on low for 8 ½ hours.
5. Stir in coconut milk and puree the soup with an immersion blender.
6. Add parsley and cook the soup for an additional 30 minutes.
7. Serve sprinkled with pumpkin seeds.

Minestrone Soup

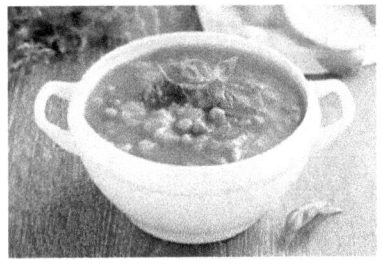

Preparation time: **10 minutes**
Cooking time**: 5 hours**
Serve: 4

Ingredients:
- 2 tablespoons coconut oil
- 2 carrots, chopped
- 2 stalks celery, chopped
- 1 onion, diced

- 2 cloves garlic, minced
- 2 sprigs rosemary, chopped
- 1 tomato, pureed (puree in a food blender)
- 1 tablespoon thyme, chopped
- 0.75lb. chopped tomatoes
- 4 cups vegetable stock
- 10oz. cooked cannellini beans
- 1oz. green peas
- 1oz. spaghetti
- 4oz. spring greens, chopped
- Salt and pepper, to taste
- 1 tablespoon extra-virgin olive oil

Instructions:
1. Heat coconut oil in a skillet over medium-high heat.
2. Add the carrots, celery, and onion. Cook stirring for 5 minutes.
3. Add garlic and herbs — Cook for 1 minute.
4. Add pureed tomato and cook for 4 minutes.
5. Transfer the mixture into the slow cooker.
6. Add vegetable stock and cook on low for 4 hours.
7. Stir in the beans, pasta, greens, and peas.
8. Season to taste with salt and pepper, and continue to cook for 30 minutes, with the lid on.
9. Serve Minestrone warm, drizzled with olive oil.

Miso Soup

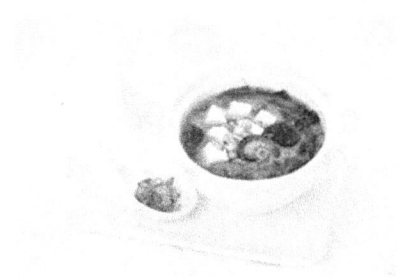

Preparation time: **10 minutes**
Cooking time: 6 hours 40 minutes
Serve: 4

Ingredients:
- 4 ½ cups water
- 3 tablespoons miso paste, white or yellow
- 8oz. extra-firm tofu, drained, cubed
- 2 spring onions, chopped
- 1 clove garlic, minced
- 0.25lb. button mushrooms
- 1 ½ cups sliced sugar peas

Instructions:
1. Pour water into slow cooker.
2. Whisk on miso paste.

3. Add tofu, mushrooms, and garlic and cover with a lid. Cook on low for 6 hours.
4. In the last 30 minutes of cooking, stir in spring onions.
5. Turn off the slow cooker and add snap peas. Let the soup rest for 10 minutes.
6. Serve warm.

Cauliflower Soup

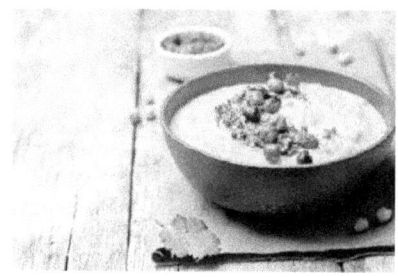

Preparation time: **10 minutes**
Cooking time: **6 hours**
Serve: 6

Ingredients:
- 1 small head cauliflower, cut into florets
- 2 cups cooked chickpeas
- 4 cloves garlic, minced
- 1 sprig thyme, chopped
- 2 small potatoes, peeled, cubed
- 4 cups vegetable stock

- Salt and pepper, to taste
- ½ teaspoon red pepper, flakes
- 1 teaspoon cumin powder
- 1 cup coconut milk

Instructions:
1. Place cauliflower, garlic, thyme, potatoes, vegetable stock, and cumin powder in a slow cooker.
2. Close with a lid and cook on low for 4-6 hours.
3. In the last 30 minutes of cooking, stir in red pepper flakes, chickpeas, and coconut milk. Cook for 30 minutes and remove from the heat.
4. Puree with an immersion blender.
5. Serve warm.

Creamy Tomato Soup

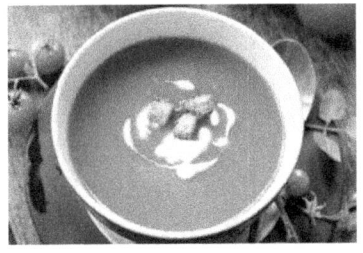

Preparation time: **20 minutes**
Cooking time: **8 hours**
Serve: 8

Ingredients:
- 3lb. ripe tomatoes
- 2 cups vegetable stock
- 1 small onion, diced
- 2 carrots, diced
- 2 cloves garlic, minced
- 2 teaspoons dried oregano
- 4 tablespoons coconut oil
- 1 cup unsweetened coconut milk
- Salt and pepper, to taste

Instructions:
1. Peel the tomatoes; make a small "x" sign at the bottom of each tomato.
2. Place the tomatoes into a large bowl and cover with boiling water. Let the tomatoes rest for 1 minute.
3. Rinse the tomatoes under cold water and peel each tomato. Chop the tomatoes afterward.
4. Place the tomatoes into a slow cooker, with the rest of the ingredients.
5. Set the slow cooker to low and cook the soup for 6-8 hours.
6. Pour ½ the soup into a food blender.
7. Blend until smooth and combine with the remaining soup or puree the soup completely with an immersion blender.
8. Serve soup warm.

Vegan Pho Soup

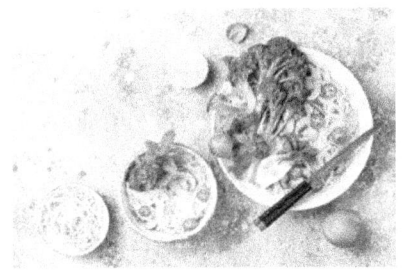

Preparation time: **10 minutes**
Cooking time: 4 hours 10 minutes
Serve: 4

Ingredients:
- 1 small onion, chopped
- 4 cloves garlic, halved
- 1-inch ginger root, peeled, thinly sliced
- 2 green chilies, sliced
- 1 teaspoon Chinese five-spice powder
- 4 cups water
- ¼ cup soy sauce or coconut aminos
- 1 tablespoon balsamic vinegar
- 1lb. whole mushrooms
- 7oz. rice noodles

Serve with:
- 6 spring onions, chopped
- 3oz. broccolini, steamed

- 2 tablespoons chopped coriander
- 1 lime, cut into wedges

Instructions:
1. Combine onion, garlic, ginger, chilies, and Chinee spice powder in a slow cooker.
2. Add water and soy sauce.
3. Add in the mushrooms.
4. Cover and cook on low for 4 hours.
5. Drain the cooked content in a bowl, collecting the cooking juices. Slice the mushrooms into thick slices.
6. Combine the stock (cooking liquid) with balsamic vinegar in a saucepot. Bring to a boil.
7. In the meantime, cook noodles according to package directions.
8. Drain the noodles and place into a bowl.
9. Top with mushrooms, spring onions, broccolini, and coriander. Ladle the stock over noodles.
10. Serve warm with lime wedges.

White Bean Soup

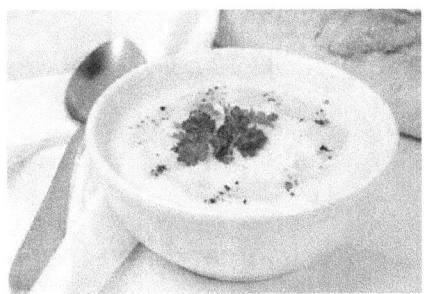

Preparation time: **10 minutes**
Cooking time: **10 hours**
Serve: 6

Ingredients:
- 1lb. Cannellini beans, soaked overnight
- ¼ cup olive oil
- 1 onion, diced
- 1 fennel bulb. trimmed, sliced
- 2 stalks celery, chopped
- 4 cloves garlic, minced
- 2 sprigs fresh rosemary, chopped
- 1 teaspoon fennel seeds
- 6 cups vegetable stock
- 1 lemon, juiced
- ¼ cup parsley, chopped
- Salt and pepper, to taste

Instructions:
1. Rinse and drain the beans. Place the beans in a slow cooker.
2. Heat olive oil in a skillet.
3. Add onion and cook stirring for 5 minutes over medium-high heat.
4. Add the fennel bulb and cook for an additional 5 minutes.
5. Add celery, garlic, rosemary, and fennel seeds. Cook for 2 minutes.
6. Transfer the mixture into the slow cooker.
7. Add vegetable stock and season to taste. Close the cooker with lid and cook the beans on low for 8-10 hours.
8. Before serving to remove the rosemary sprigs. Puree the soup with an immersion blender and stir in lemon juice and parsley.
9. Serve.

Split Pea Soup

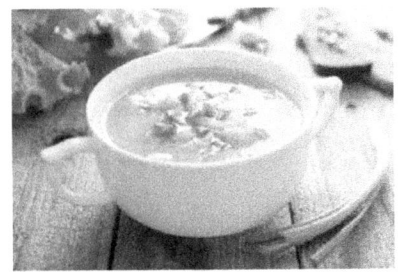

Preparation time: **10 minutes**
Cooking time: **6 hours**
Serve: 4

Ingredients:
- 2 cups split pea soup
- 3 carrots, chopped
- 1 onion, diced
- 2 stalks celery, chopped
- 1 shallot, chopped
- 2 cloves garlic, minced
- 1 bay leaf
- 4 cups vegetable stock
- ½ cup unsweetened coconut milk
- Salt and pepper, to taste

Instructions:
1. Rinse the split peas and place in a slow cooker.

2. Add carrots, onion, celery, shallot, garlic, bay leaf, and vegetable stock.
3. Cover and cook on low for 6 hours.
4. In the last 30 minutes of cooking, stir in coconut milk.
5. Puree the soup after 6 hours with an immersion blender.
6. Reheat soup for 10 minutes on low.
7. Serve the soup warm.
8. You can serve the soup with toasted bread.

Kidney Beans And Wild Mushroom Soup

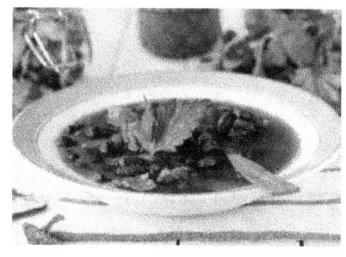

Preparation time: **10 minutes**
Cooking time:**6 hours**
Serve: 6

Ingredients:
- 1lb. wild mushrooms, cleaned and torn into pieces
- ½ onion, sliced
- 4 cloves garlic, minced

- 4 cups vegetable stock
- 1 ½ cups cooked kidney beans
- 1 sprig rosemary
- Salt and pepper, to taste
- ¼ cup chopped parsley

Instructions:
1. Combine mushrooms, onion, garlic, and vegetable stock in a slow cooker.
2. Season to taste and add rosemary.
3. Cover the slow cooker with lid. Cook the mushrooms on high for 3 ½ hours.
4. Remove the rosemary and add beans.
5. Continue to cook on high for 30 minutes.
6. Serve warm, sprinkled with chopped parsley.

Creamy Broccoli Soup

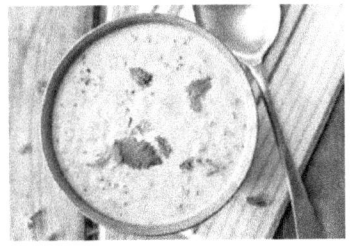

Preparation time: **10 minutes**
Cooking time: **6 hours**
Serve: 4

Ingredients:
- 2 tablespoons olive oil
- 1 onion, diced
- 2 cloves garlic, minced
- 2 carrots, chopped
- 2 cups vegetable stock
- 4 cups broccoli florets, stems removed
- 1 cup cashews, soaked overnight, rinsed and drained
- 1 cup water
- ½ cup nutritional yeast
- ½ teaspoon smoked paprika powder
- ¼ teaspoon mustard powder
- Salt and pepper, to taste
- ¼ cup almond milk
- ½ lemon, juiced

Instructions:
1. Set your slow cooker to low.
2. Heat olive oil in a skillet.
3. Add onion and carrots and cook stirring for 5 minutes over medium-high heat.
4. Add garlic and spices and cook until very fragrant.
5. Transfer the veggies into the slow cooker.
6. Add vegetable stock and close with the lid. Cook the broccoli on low for 6 hours.
7. In the meantime, rinse and drain cashews.

8. Place the cashews in a food blender. Add nutritional yeast, almond milk, and water. Blend until smooth.
9. Pour the cashew mixture into the broccoli 30 minutes before cooking is done.
10. Continue to cook for 30 minutes.
11. Once done, puree the soup with an immersion blender. Adjust the seasoning and stir in lemon juice.
12. Serve soup warm.

Slow Cooker Main Courses

Mediterranean Stuffed Peppers

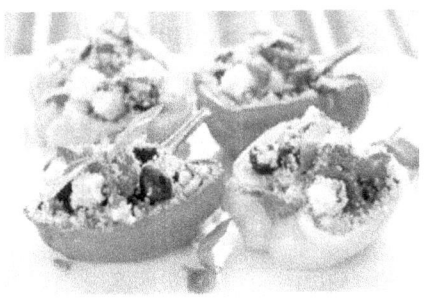

Preparation time: **15 minutes**
Cooking time: **6 hours**
Serve: 4

Ingredients:
- 4 bell peppers, any color
- ¾ cup quinoa

- 1 cup pureed tomatoes (puree in a food blender)
- 4 sun-dried tomatoes, packed in oil, chopped
- ½ cup black olives, sliced
- 4oz. firm tofu, cubed
- 2 tablespoons lemon juice
- 1 teaspoon dried basil
- Salt and pepper, to taste
- 2 tablespoons toasted pine nuts
- Chopped parsley, to serve with

Instructions:
1. Cut off the bell pepper tops and remove inner membrane and seeds.
2. In a large mixing bowl, combine quinoa, tomato sauce, sun-dried tomatoes, and olives.
3. Toss the tofu with lemon juice and basil and add to the quinoa. Season with salt and pepper, to taste.
4. Stuff the peppers with prepared mixture.
5. Pour ½ cup water into slow cooker.
6. Place the peppers into the slow cooker, so they are sitting in the water.
7. Close the cooker with a lid.
8. Cook the bell peppers on low setting for 6 hours.
9. Remove the bell peppers from the slow cooker and cut in half.
10. Sprinkle with parsley and pine nuts.
11. Serve.

Pasta With Rich Sauce

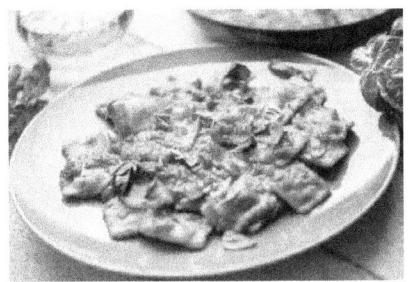

Preparation time: **10 minutes**
Cooking time: **6 hours**
Serve: 4

Ingredients:

Sauce:
- 0.75lb. ripe tomatoes, chopped
- 1 red bell pepper, seeded, chopped
- 6 cloves garlic, minced
- 1 teaspoon dried basil
- Salt and pepper, to taste
- 1 cup raw cashews, rinsed

Pasta:
- 12oz. Vegan pasta or zoodles

Instructions:
1. Combine the sauce ingredients in a slow cooker.

2. Close with a lid and cook on low setting for 6 hours.
3. Just before serving cook the pasta according to package directions.
4. Puree the sauce with an immersion blender or food blender.
5. Serve over pasta and serve.

Indian Stuffed Pancakes

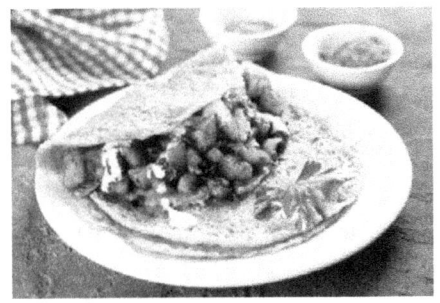

Preparation time: 10 minutes
Cooking time: 5 hours
Serve: 4

Ingredients:

Pancakes:
- ½ tablespoon cumin seeds powder
- 5oz. chickpea flour
- Salt and pepper, to taste
- 1 chili pepper, chopped
- 2 ½ cups almond milk
- Coconut oil, for frying

Filling:
- 1lb. gold potatoes, cubed
- 0.25lb. carrots, cubed
- ½ cup vegetable stock
- 1 teaspoon curry powder
- Salt and pepper, to taste

- 2 tablespoons chopped parsley

Instructions:
1. Make the filling; combine all the filling ingredients in a slow cooker.
2. Cover and cook on low for 5 hours.
3. Make the pancakes; start preparing pancakes 30 minutes before the filling is cooked.
4. Combine the pancake ingredients in a food blender. Blend until smooth. Let the batter rest for 10 minutes. Add more almond milk if needed as the batter needs to be runny.
5. Brush large skillet over coconut oil and heat over medium-high heat.
6. Pour less than ½ cup of the batter into the skillet and with a swirl motion distribute the batter evenly over the skillet bottom. Cook the pancakes for 2 minutes per side.
7. Spread some of the fillings over the pancake. Fold the pancake over filling and serve.

Spiced Kofta In Sauce

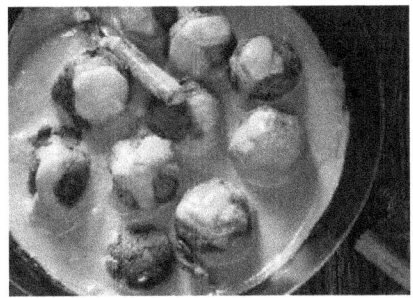

Preparation time: 15 minutes
Cooking time: 5 ½ hours
Serve: 6

Ingredients:

Kofta:
- 2 cups mashed potatoes or leftover potatoes
- 1lb. extra-firm tofu, drained
- ½ cup arrowroot starch or cornstarch
- Salt and pepper, to taste
- 1 tablespoon lemon juice
- ¼ cup chopped parsley
- 1 ½ teaspoons garam masala
- Coconut oil, for frying

Sauce:
- 1 onion, chopped
- 6 ripe tomatoes, chopped

- 4 cloves garlic, minced
- ¼ cup raw cashews, rinsed
- Salt and pepper, to taste
- 2 teaspoons curry powder
- 2 cups unsweetened coconut milk
- ½ teaspoon cayenne pepper

Instructions:
1. Make the sauce; combine all the sauce ingredients in a slow cooker.
2. Cover and cook on low for 5 hours.
3. 30 minutes before the sauce is done, make the kofta.
4. Place mashed potatoes in a bowl. Add tofu and mash with a fork.
5. Add starch, salt, pepper, lemon juice, parsley, and garam masala. Stir to combine.
6. Add more starch if needed. Shape the mixture into 1-inch or walnut size balls.
7. Heat approx. 2 tablespoons of coconut oil in a skillet over medium-high heat.
8. Add prepared kofta and cook in the heated oil for 7-8 minutes or until browned on all sides. Remove from the heat.
9. Puree the sauce with an immersion blender or food blender. Gently add the kofta.
10. Cover and continue to cook on low for 30 minutes.
11. Serve warm with quinoa or rice.

Vegan Greek Moussaka

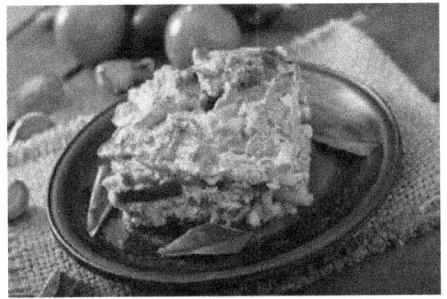

Preparation time: 30 minutes

Cooking time: 5 hours 20 minutes

Serve: 6

Ingredients:
- 1 tablespoon coconut oil
- 1 large potato, peeled, thinly sliced
- 1 eggplant, trimmed, thinly sliced
- Salt and pepper, to taste
- 1lb. brown mushrooms, finely chopped
- 1 onion, chopped
- 2 cloves garlic, minced
- ½ cup chopped parsley
- ½ cup chopped black olives
- ½ cup vegetable stock
- 4 tomatoes, chopped
- 2 ½ cups unsweetened almond milk

- ½ cup all-purpose flour
- ½ teaspoon turmeric
- 2 tablespoons nutritional yeast

Instructions:

1. Grease your slow cooker with some of the coconut oil.
2. Arrange the potato slices in the slow cooker, so the bottom is covered.
3. Sprinkle the eggplant with salt and place aside for 15 minutes.
4. In the meantime, heat the remaining coconut oil in a skillet.
5. Add mushrooms, onion, and garlic. Cook stirring for 5 minutes.
6. Add parsley, vegetable stock, olives, and tomatoes. Simmer for 10 minutes.
7. Transfer half the mushroom mixture into the slow cooker. Top with eggplant slices and cover with the remaining mushrooms. Cover and cook on low for 3 hours.
8. In the meantime, whisk 1 cup almond milk with flour.
9. Set the mixture over medium-high heat and bring to a gentle boil.
10. Reduce heat and stir in the remaining milk, turmeric, and nutritional yeast. Cook until the sauce is gently thickened.

11. Pour the mixture over moussaka and continue to cook on low for 2 hours.
12. Let the moussaka rest for 30 minutes before serving.

Seitan Eggplant Stew

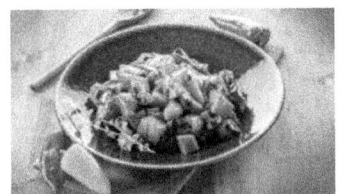

Preparation time: **10 minutes**
Cooking time: 6 hours 10 minutes
Serve: 6

Ingredients:
- 1 tablespoon coconut oil
- 1 onion, chopped
- 4 cloves garlic
- 10oz. seitan, cubed
- 1 cup yellow split peas
- 2 red bell peppers, seeded, sliced
- 6 cups water
- 1 large eggplant, trimmed, cubed

- 2 tablespoons pomegranate molasses
- Salt and pepper, to taste
- 1 teaspoon smoked paprika
- 1 teaspoon cumin powder
- 1 teaspoon coriander powder
- ½ teaspoon cayenne pepper

Instructions:
1. Heat coconut oil in a skillet over medium-high heat. Add seitan and cook for 2 minutes per side. Place the seitan aside.
2. In the same skillet cook onion with spices and garlic until very fragrant.
3. Transfer into the slow cooker.
4. Add split peas and water — cover and cook on low for 4 hours.
5. Add eggplants, bell peppers, and seitan.
6. Continue to cook for an additional 2 hours.
7. Serve stew warm.

Vegetable Lasagna

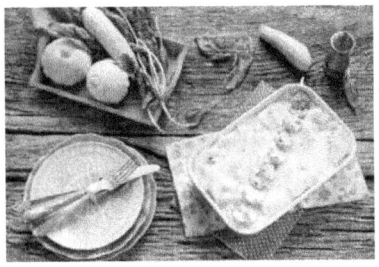

Preparation time: **20 minutes**
Cooking time: 3 hours 20 minutes
Serve: 6

Ingredients:
- 1 tablespoon coconut oil
- 2 large onions, diced
- 4 cloves garlic, minced
- 1.5lb. zucchini, chopped
- 1 red bell pepper, seeded, sliced
- 1 yellow bell pepper, seeded, sliced
- 1 green bell pepper, seeded, sliced
- 1lb. chopped tomatoes
- ½ cup fresh basil
- 1 large eggplant, sliced
- 9 Vegan lasagna sheets
- Salt and pepper, to taste

Instructions:

1. Heat olive oil in a skillet.
2. Add onions and cook stirring for 5 minutes over medium-high heat.
3. Add garlic and cook for 1 minute.
4. Add zucchini, and bell peppers. Stir to combine.
5. Add the tomatoes and basil. Cook for 5 minutes.
6. Arrange the eggplant slices in the slow cooker.
7. Top with 3 lasagna sheets.
8. Add 1/3 of the mixture. Repeat layers until you have used all the filling and lasagna sheets.
9. Cover and cook on high for 6 hours.
10. Serve warm.

Burger "Steak" Balls

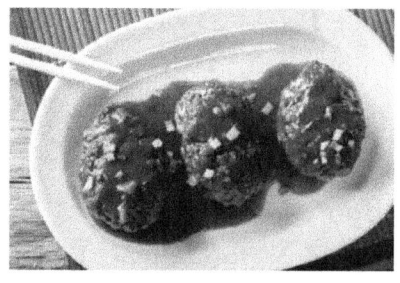

Preparation time: **15 minutes**
Cooking time: 4 hours 10 minutes
Serve: 4

Ingredients:

"Burger" balls:
- 2 cups cooked kidney beans
- 1 cup cooked quinoa
- 2 tablespoons tomato paste, organic
- 1 onion, finely chopped
- ½ teaspoon mustard powder
- ½ teaspoon garlic powder
- 1 teaspoon celery flakes
- 1 pinch nutmeg
- 1 tablespoon coconut oil
- 2 spring onions, chopped

Sauce:
- 1 tablespoon olive oil
- 1 onion, chopped
- 2 cloves garlic, minced
- 4 Roma tomatoes, chopped
- 2 beefsteak tomatoes, pureed
- ½ teaspoon dried basil
- 1 chili pepper, seeded, chopped
- Salt and pepper, to taste
- ¼ cup vegetable stock
- 2 tablespoons coconut aminos or soy sauce

Ingredients:
1. Make the sauce; heat olive oil in a skillet. Add onions, garlic, and chili pepper. Cook until fragrant for 4-5 minutes.
2. Transfer the rest of the ingredients.

3. Cover and cook on low for 3 hours.
4. In the meantime, make the balls; mash the kidney beans in a bowl.
5. Add the rest of the ingredients, except the oil, and stir with a fork to combine.
6. Shape the mixture into 8 balls.
7. Heat coconut oil in a skillet over medium-high heat. Add the balls and cook until browned on all sides.
8. Remove the lid from the slow cooker. Puree the sauce with an immersion blender.
9. Place in the balls and cover. Continue to cook on low for 1 hour.
10. Serve "steak" balls warm with sauce and sprinkled with chopped spring onion.

Mushroom Tempeh Stroganoff

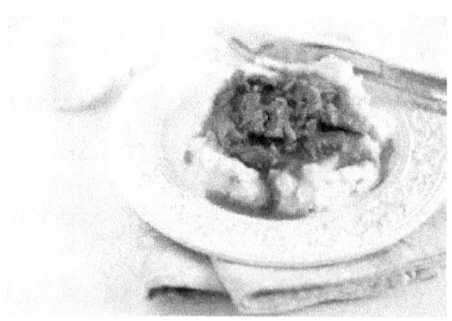

Preparation time: 10 minutes + inactive time
Cooking time: **8 hours**

Serve: 4

Ingredients:
- 10oz. tempeh
- 0.5lb. sliced mushrooms
- 2 large onions, sliced
- 4 cloves garlic, minced
- 3 ½ cups vegetable stock
- 2 tablespoons coconut aminos or soy sauce
- 2/3 cup cashew cream
- 1 teaspoon smoked paprika
- Salt and pepper, to taste
- ½ cup chopped parsley

Serve with:
- Mashed potatoes

Instructions:
1. Cut tempeh and place into steaming basket.
2. Set the tempeh over 2-inches of simmering water. Cover with lid and steam for 10 minutes.
3. Refrigerate the tempeh till morning.
4. When ready to cook; combine tempeh, mushrooms, onions, garlic, vegetable stock, spices, and coconut aminos in a slow cooker.
5. Cover and cook on low for 8 hours.
6. Few minutes before the cooking is done, stir in cashew cream and parsley.
7. Serve stroganoff over mashed potatoes.

Tofu Veggie Stew

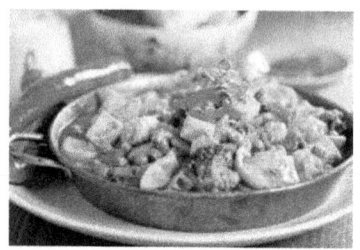

Preparation time: **10 minutes**
Cooking time: **6 hours**
Serve: 6

Ingredients:
- 1lb. extra-firm tofu, cubed
- 2 cups cauliflower florets
- 2 cups broccoli florets
- 1 cup frozen peas
- 1 red bell pepper, seeded, sliced
- 2 white potatoes, peeled, cubed
- Salt and pepper, to taste
- 1 cup vegetable stock
- 1 chili pepper, seeded, chopped
- 1 onion, diced
- 1 bay leaf
- 1 teaspoon paprika powder
- 1 teaspoon fresh thyme
- 1 teaspoon chopped basil

Instructions:
1. Combine tofu, cauliflower, broccoli, peas, bell pepper, potatoes, vegetable stock, chili pepper, onion, bay leaf and paprika in a slow cooker.
2. Cover and cook on low for 6 hours.
3. Serve stew warm with cooked rice.

Okra Gumbo

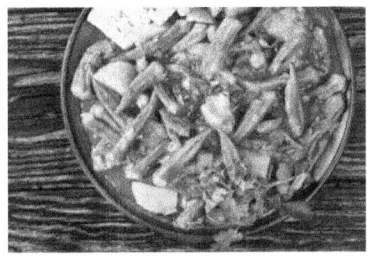

Preparation time: **10 minutes**
Cooking time: **6 hours**
Serve: 6

Ingredients:
- 1 onion, chopped
- 3 cloves garlic, minced
- 2 stalks celery, chopped
- 2 carrots, peeled, chopped
- 3 cups vegetable stock
- 4 tomatoes, chopped
- 2 cups frozen okra

- ½ cup pureed tomatoes (just puree in a food blender)
- 2 white potatoes, peeled, cubed
- 1 cup sliced mushrooms
- Salt and pepper, to taste
- 2 teaspoons Cajun seasoning
- 3 tablespoons chopped parsley

Instructions:
1. Combine onion, garlic, celery, carrots, vegetable stock, tomatoes, okra, pureed tomatoes, white potatoes, mushrooms, salt, pepper, and Cajun seasoning in a slow cooker.
2. Cover with lid and cook on low for 6 hours.
3. Stir in parsley just before serving.
4. Serve gumbo warm with cooked brown rice.

Vegan Palak Paneer

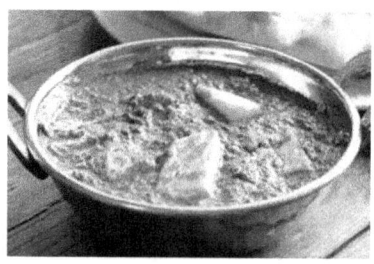

Preparation time: **10 minutes**
Cooking time: 4 hours 45 minutes

Serve: 6

Ingredients:
- 4 cloves garlic
- 2-inch piece ginger, minced
- 4 tomatoes, pureed (just puree in a food blender)
- 1 tablespoon ground coriander
- 1 tablespoon Garam masala
- ½ tablespoon cumin powder
- Salt and pepper, to taste
- 4 cups spinach
- 2 cups unsweetened coconut milk
- 12oz. extra-firm tofu, cubed
- 2 tablespoons coconut oil
- ½ cup frozen peas

Instructions:
1. Combine garlic, ginger, pureed tomatoes, coriander, Garam masala, cumin, and coconut milk in a slow cooker.
2. Cover and cook on low for 4 hours.
3. Heat coconut oil in a skillet over medium-high heat. Season tofu with salt and pepper.
4. Cook the tofu in heated oil for 3 minutes per side.
5. At 3 hours and 30 minutes add spinach and peas.
6. Continue to cook for 30 minutes. Remove the lid and puree the spinach and peas with an immersion blender.
7. Add tofu and continue to cook for 15 minutes.

8. Serve warm with cooked rice.

Lentils Cauliflower Curry

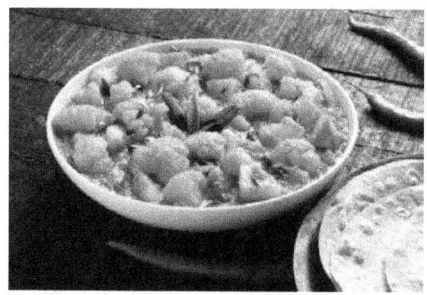

Preparation time: **10 minutes**
Cooking time: **8 hours**
Serve: 6

Ingredients:
- 1 cup red lentils, rinsed
- 2 white potatoes, peeled, cubed
- 1 small head cauliflower, cut into florets
- 1 onion, thinly sliced
- 3 cloves garlic, minced
- ½ tablespoon minced ginger
- 1 tablespoon red curry paste
- 2 tomatoes, pureed (puree in a food blender)
- ¼ cup coconut milk

- ½ teaspoon turmeric
- ¼ teaspoon cayenne pepper
- ¼ teaspoon ground cumin seeds
- ¼ teaspoon ground coriander seeds
- Salt and pepper, to taste
- ¼ cup chopped cilantro

Serve with:
- Cooked brown rice

Instructions:
1. Combine rinsed red lentils, potatoes, and cauliflower in a slow cooker.
2. Add the spices and pour over pureed tomatoes.
3. Cover with lid and cook on low for 7-8 hours.
4. Few minutes before serving, stir in coconut milk.
5. Serve curry over rice.

Pasta Puttanesca

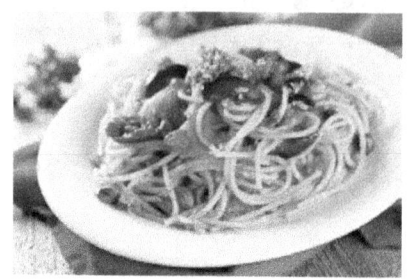

Preparation time: **10 minutes**
Cooking time: **5 hours**
Serve: 4

Ingredients:
- 1.5lb. Ripe tomatoes, peeled*
- 0.5lb. mushrooms, coarse chopped
- ½ cup black olives pitted
- 2 tablespoons capers, drained
- 1 onion, chopped
- 2 cloves garlic, minced
- 1 tablespoon balsamic vinegar
- Salt and pepper, to taste
- Fresh basil, chopped

Serve with:
- 8oz. Vegan spaghetti

Instructions:
1. Combine tomatoes, mushrooms, olives, capers, onion, garlic, and balsamic vinegar in a slow cooker.
2. Season to taste and close with the lid.
3. Cook on low for 5 hours.
4. Just before serving, cook the pasta according to package instructions.
5. Serve puttanesca sauce over pasta.

*NOTE: Peel the tomatoes by cutting an "x" sign at the bottom of each tomato. Place the tomatoes in a large bowl and cover with boiling water. Allow to stand for 30 seconds. Rinse the tomatoes under cold water and peel the skin. Chop before use.

Lentils Veggie Rolls

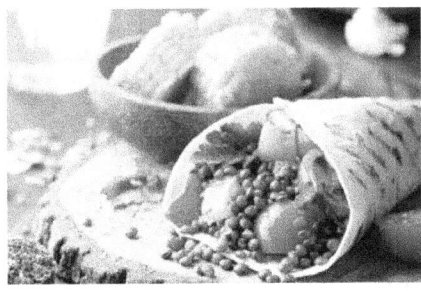

Preparation time: **15 minutes**

Cooking time: **4 hours**
Serve: 6

Ingredients:
- 1 cup brown lentils, rinsed
- 1 cup brown mushrooms, chopped
- 1 red bell pepper, seeded, sliced
- 1 yellow bell pepper, seeded, sliced
- 3 cups vegetable stock
- 1 cup frozen corn
- 1 onion, diced
- 2 cloves garlic, minced
- ¼ cup chopped parsley
- Salt and pepper to taste
- 1 teaspoon chili powder
- 1 teaspoon cumin powder
- 1 teaspoon coriander powder

Serve with:
- 6 corn tortilla wraps
- 6 cherry tomatoes, chopped
- 1 large avocado, chopped
- 1 jalapeno, seeded, chopped
- Salt and pepper, to taste

Instructions:
1. Make the lentils filling; combine lentil, mushrooms, red bell pepper, yellow bell pepper, vegetable stock,

corn, onion, garlic, parsley, salt, pepper, chili, cumin, and coriander.
2. Cover and cook on low for 4 hours.
3. To serve; heat tortillas in a microwave.
4. Combine tomatoes, avocado, jalapeno, lime juice, salt and pepper in a bowl.
5. Fill each tortilla with lentils and top with tomato mixture.
6. Roll and serve.

White Bean Quinoa Chili

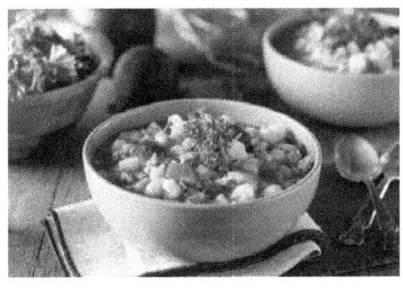

Preparation time: **10 minutes**
Cooking time: **8 hours**
Serve: 4

Ingredients:
- 1 onion, chopped
- 1 cup white beans, soaked overnight, rinsed and drained

- 1 cup corn
- 1 cup quinoa
- 4oz. silken tofu, pureed (puree in a food blender)
- 2 green bell peppers, seeded, chopped
- 1lb. chopped tomatoes
- 3 cups vegetable stock
- 2 tablespoons chili powder
- Salt and pepper, to taste
- ¼ cup chopped cilantro
- 1 avocado, chopped, to serve with

Instructions:
1. Combine onion, white beans, corn, quinoa, tofu, green bell peppers, chopped tomatoes, vegetable stock, chili, salt, and pepper, to taste.
2. Cover with lid and cook on low for 8 hours.
3. If needed add some water during the cooking time.
4. In the last minutes of cooking, stir in cilantro.
5. Serve chili warm, topped with chopped avocado.

Lasagna Rolls

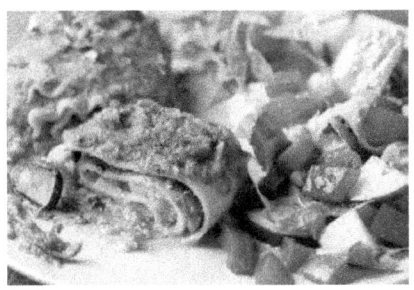

Preparation time: 20 minutes
Cooking time: 4 hours
Serve: 8

Ingredients:
- 8 Vegan lasagna sheets
- 1.5lb tomatoes, peeled*
- 1 jalapeno pepper, seeded
- ½ cup fresh basil
- 3 cloves garlic, peeled
- Salt and pepper, to taste
- 1 zucchini, grated, water squeezed out
- 1 cup sliced mushrooms
- 12oz. extra-firm tofu, drained
- ¾ cup hummus
- ¼ cup nutritional yeast

Instructions:

1. Cook the lasagna sheets according to package directions.
2. In the meantime, combine tomatoes, jalapeno, basil, garlic, and salt and pepper, to taste in a food blender.
3. Pour ¾ cup of the tomato sauce in a slow cooker.
4. Heat coconut oil in a skillet. Add mushrooms and zucchini. Cook for 5 minutes.
5. Mash the tofu with hummus in a bowl. Stir in mushrooms and zucchini.
6. Lay cooked zucchini sheets on a baking paper.
7. Place around ¼ cup of the tofu mixture over the lasagna sheet.
8. Roll the lasagna sheet and place in a slow cooker, seam side down.
9. Repeat with the remaining ingredients.
10. Pour the remaining tomato sauce over the lasagna rolls. Cover and cook on low for 4 hours.
11. Serve warm with fresh salad.

*NOTE: Peel the tomatoes by cutting an "x" sign at the bottom of each tomato. Place the tomatoes in a large bowl and cover with boiling water. Allow to stand for 30 seconds. Rinse the tomatoes under cold water and peel the skin. Chop before use.

Lentils Sweet Potato Stew

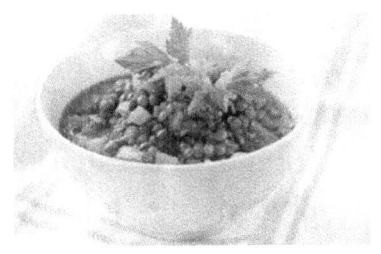

Preparation time: **10 minutes**
Cooking time: 8 hours 15 minutes
Serve: 6

Ingredients:
- 1 large onion, diced
- 1 ½ tablespoon coconut oil
- 1-inch piece ginger, minced
- 2 cloves garlic, minced
- 6 tomatoes, chopped
- 1 sweet potato, peeled, cubed
- 2 ½ cups vegetable stock
- 1 ½ cups water
- 1 ½ cups dried lentils, rinsed
- Salt and pepper, to taste
- 3oz. chopped green chilies
- 1 ½ teaspoon coriander powder
- 1 ½ teaspoon powder
- ½ cup unsweetened coconut milk
- 1 tablespoon cornstarch

Instructions:
1. Heat coconut oil in a large skillet.
2. Add onions and cook for 5 minutes over medium-high heat.
3. Add ginger and garlic. Cook 1 minute. Add tomatoes and simmer until they release juices.
4. Transfer the onion mixture into a slow cooker.
5. Add sweet potato, lentils, spices, stock, and water — season to taste with salt and pepper.
6. Cover and cook on low for 8 hours or until the lentils are tender.
7. Combine coconut milk and cornstarch until smooth.
8. In the last minutes of cooking, stir in coconut milk mixture.
9. Cook for at least 5 minutes.
10. Serve stew warm.

Something Like Risotto

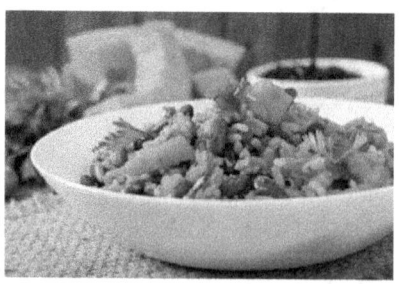

Preparation time: **10 minutes**

Cooking time: **3 hours**
Serve: 4

Ingredients:
- 1 tablespoon olive oil
- 1 cup Arborio rice
- 1lb. cubed pumpkin
- 1 cup cooked kidney beans
- 2 cups vegetable stock
- 1 cinnamons tock, broken in half
- 4 black peppercorns
- 1 pinch nutmeg
- 2 tablespoons chopped parsley
- Salt, to taste
- 1 tablespoon pine nuts

Instructions:
1. Heat olive oil in a skillet over medium-high heat.
2. Add rice and cook until translucent.
3. Transfer the rice into the slow cooker.
4. Add pumpkin, kidney beans, vegetable stock, cinnamon, nutmeg, peppercorns, and salt.
5. Close the cooker with lid and cook on low for 3 hours.
6. After three hours, remove cinnamon stick, and stir in parsley.
7. Serve warm, sprinkled with pine nuts.

Sweet And Sour Tofu With Quinoa

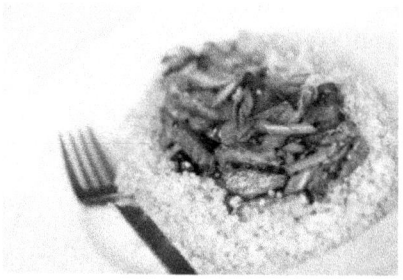

Preparation time: **10 minutes**
Cooking time: **6 hours**
Serve: **4**

Ingredients:
- 1lb. extra-firm tofu, drained, pressed, sliced
- 1 cup fresh pineapple juice
- ¼ cup rice vinegar
- 2 tablespoons balsamic vinegar
- 3 tablespoons agave
- Salt and pepper, to taste
- 2 spring onions, sliced

Quinoa:
- 1 cup quinoa
- 2 cups vegetable stock or water
- Salt, to taste

Instructions:
1. In a bowl, combine pineapple juice, vinegar, balsamic vinegar, and agave.
2. Add it to slow cooker along with sliced tofu.
3. Cook the tofu on low for 6 hours.
4. Make the quinoa; cook quinoa in simmering vegetable stock for 15 minutes.
5. Remove from the heat and allow to stand for 5 minutes.
6. Serve quinoa, topped with tofu and cooking juices.
7. Finish off with the sliced spring onions.

Vegetables, Grains, And Beans Salads

Quinoa With Grilled Pineapple

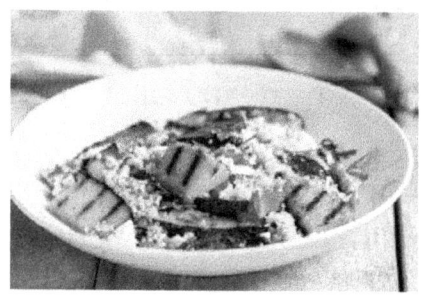

Preparation time: **10 minutes**
Cooking time: **4 hours**
Serve: 4

Ingredients:
- 1 cup quinoa
- 1 ½ cups water
- Salt, to taste

Additional:
- 1 cup sliced pineapples
- 2 small beets, peeled, sliced
- 1 tablespoon olive oil
- 2 tablespoons chopped parsley
- 2 tablespoons lemon juice

Instructions:

1. Combine quinoa, water, and salt to taste in a slow cooker.
2. Cover and cook on low for 4 hours.
3. Before serving; brush the pineapple and beet with olive oil.
4. Grill the pineapple and beets for 4 minutes per side over the grill or in the grill pan.
5. Toss the quinoa with chopped parsley, lemon juice, pineapple, and beets.
6. Serve warm.

Delicious Ratatouille

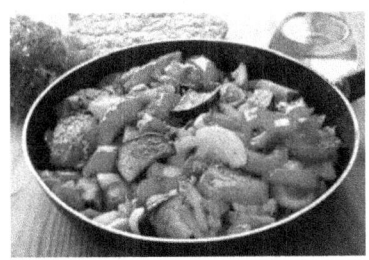

Preparation time: **10 minutes**
Cooking time: **6 hours**
Serve: **6**

Ingredients:
- 3 tablespoons olive oil
- 1 onion, diced

- 3 cloves garlic, minced
- 0.75lb. eggplants, sliced
- 0.75lb. zucchinis, sliced
- 3 ripe tomatoes, sliced
- 1 red bell pepper, seeded, sliced
- Salt and pepper, to taste
- 3 tablespoons chopped basil leaves

Instructions:
1. Heat 1 tablespoon olive oil in a skillet.
2. Add onion and cook stirring for 20 minutes over medium-low heat or until browned.
3. Stir in garlic and remove from the heat.
4. Add eggplants, zucchini, tomatoes, and bell pepper into the slow cooker.
5. Drizzle the vegetables with remaining olive oil.
6. Scatter browned onions and garlic over veggies.
7. Season the ratatouille with salt and pepper, and close with the lid.
8. Cook on low for 5-6 hours.
9. Sprinkle the ratatouille with basil before serving.

Baked Beans

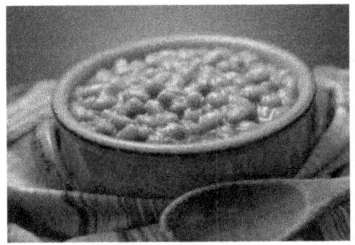

Preparation time: **10 minutes**
Cooking time: **10 hours**
Serve: 8

Ingredients:
- 1lb. dried navy beans, soaked overnight
- 1 onion, chopped
- 3 cloves garlic, minced
- 3 cups pureed tomatoes (puree in a food blender)
- 1/3 cup maple syrup
- 2 tablespoon molasses
- ¼ cup raw cider vinegar
- Salt and pepper, to taste
- 2 teaspoons mustard powder
- 1 large bay leaf
- 1 sprig rosemary, chopped
- 1 teaspoon cumin powder
- 1 tablespoon smoked paprika
- 1 cup water

Instructions:
1. Drain beans and rinse under water.
2. Place the beans in a slow cooker, along with onion, garlic, tomatoes, maple syrup, molasses, vinegar, mustard powder, bay leaf, rosemary, smoked paprika, and water.
3. Season to taste and close with the lid.
4. Cook the beans on low for 8-10 hours.
5. Serve beans warm.

Chickpeas Salad

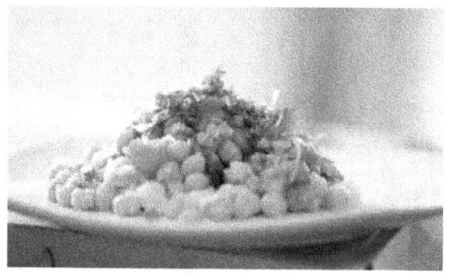

Preparation time: **10 minutes**
Cooking time: **3 hours**
Serve: **4**

Ingredients:

- ½ cup dried chickpeas, soaked overnight, rinsed and drained
- 2 cups water
- Salt, to taste

Additional:
- 2 tomatoes, chopped
- ½ cup parsley, chopped
- 2 tablespoons lemon juice
- 2 tablespoons extra-virgin olive oil
- Salt and pepper, to taste

Instructions:
1. Make the chickpeas; place the chickpeas in a slow cooker.
2. If you have not pre-soaked the chickpeas, make sure you rinse them well and remove any dirt.
3. In that case, increase cooking time for an additional hour.
4. Add water and season to taste with salt.
5. Close with a lid and cook on high for 3 hours.
6. Assemble; drain the chickpeas and place into a bowl.
7. Toss the chickpeas with tomatoes, parsley, lemon juice, oil, and salt and pepper.
8. Serve.

Quinoa Pilaf

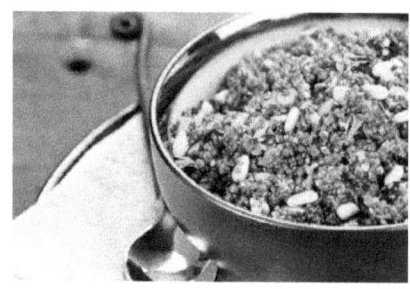

Preparation time: **10 minutes**
Cooking time: **5 hours**
Serve: 6

Ingredients:
- 1 onion, chopped
- ¾ cup fresh cranberries
- 1/3 cup wild rice
- 1 cup quinoa
- 2 cups vegetable stock
- 2 tablespoons fresh orange juice
- Salt and pepper, to taste
- 2 tablespoons pine nuts
- ½ cup chopped parsley
- Salt and pepper, to taste

Instructions:

1. Place onion, cranberries, wild rice, quinoa, vegetable stock, orange juice, salt, and pepper in a slow cooker.
2. Stir gently and close with a lid.
3. Cook the pilaf on low setting for 5 hours.
4. Once cooked the quinoa should be fluffy.
5. Remove the pilaf from the cooker and place into a bowl.
6. Sprinkle with pine nuts and parsley.
7. Serve warm.

Maple Glazed Carrots

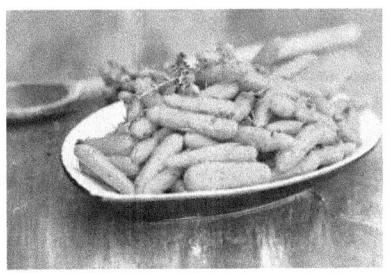

Preparation time: **10 minutes**
Cooking time: **7 hours**
Serve: 6

Ingredients:
- 2lb. baby carrots, cleaned
- 4 tablespoons coconut oil
- 2 tablespoons maple syrup

- 1 tablespoon coconut sugar
- 1 teaspoon balsamic vinegar
- Salt and pepper, to taste
- ½ teaspoon garlic powder
- ¼ teaspoon mustard powder
- 1 ½ tablespoons cornstarch
- 1 ½ tablespoons water

Instructions:
1. In a mixing bowl, combine coconut oil, maple syrup, coconut sugar, garlic powder, and mustard powder.
2. In a separate bowl, whisk water and cornstarch. Whisk in the maple syrup mixture.
3. Place the carrots in a slow cooker.
4. Pour over the maple mixture and sprinkle with salt and pepper.
5. Cover the slow cooker with lid and cook on low for 6-7 hours.
6. Serve carrots at room temperature.
7. You can serve as a side dish or puree and use for soups.

Wheat Berries Bean Salad

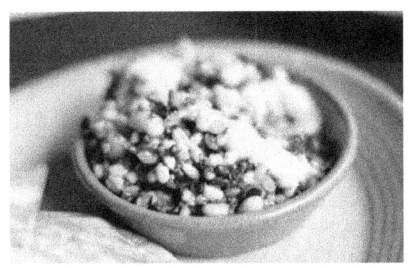

Preparation time: **10 minutes**
Cooking time: **8 hours**
Serve: **6**

Ingredients:
- 2/3 cups wheat berries
- 4 cups water
- ½ cup white beans, soaked overnight
- 1 cup frozen bob
- ¼ cup black quinoa
- 1 bay leaf
- Salt and pepper, to taste

Dressing:
- ½ cup olive oil
- ¼ cup lemon juice
- 1 tablespoon raw cider vinegar
- Salt and pepper, to taste

Instructions:

1. Combine wheat berries, water, beans, bay leaf, and salt and pepper in a slow cooker.
2. Cover and cook on low for 4 hours.
3. Add quinoa and continue to cook for an additional 4 hours.
4. In the last 30 minutes of cooking, add frozen bob.
5. Make the dressing by whisking all the ingredients together.
6. Serve salad in a large bowl. Drizzle the salad with dressing.
7. Serve as a salad or side dish.

Mexican Salad

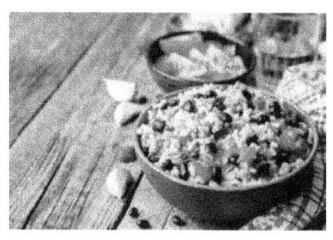

Preparation time: **10 minutes**
Cooking time: **8 hours**
Serve: 4

Ingredients:
- ½ cup black beans, soaked overnight
- 1 cup rice, rinsed

- 2 cups water
- 2 tomatoes, chopped
- 1 jalapeno, chopped
- ¼ cup chopped coriander
- Salt and pepper, to taste
- 2 tablespoon lime juice
- 2 shallots, chopped

Instructions:
1. Rinse and drain black beans. Place the beans in a slow cooker.
2. Add water and cook on low for 5 hours.
3. Add rice and more water if needed. Continue to cook on low for 3 hours.
4. Once the beans and rice are cooked, drain any liquid and transfer into a bowl.
5. While still warm, combine with chopped tomato, jalapeno, coriander, salt, pepper, lemon juice, and shallots. Toss to combine and serve.

Fresh Salad With Quinoa

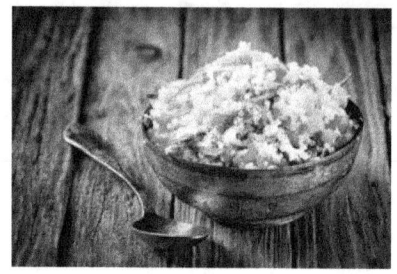

Preparation time: **10 minutes**
Cooking time: **4 hours**
Serve: 4

Ingredients:
- 1 cup quinoa
- 1 ½ cups water
- Salt and pepper, to taste

Additional:
- 1 red onion, sliced
- 1 red bell pepper, seeded, chopped
- 1 tomato, seeded, chopped
- 1 yellow bell pepper, seeded, chopped
- 1 cup sliced green beans
- 3 tablespoons extra-virgin olive oil
- 2 tablespoons lemon juice
- Salt and pepper, to taste

Instructions:
1. Rinse quinoa and drain.
2. Place the quinoa in a slow cooker along with water and salt to taste.
3. Cover and cook on low for 4 hours.
4. Once the quinoa is cooked, fluff it with a fork.
5. Steam the green beans in a steaming basket positioned over 2-inches simmering water.
6. Place the quinoa into a bowl.,
7. Add in steamed beans, sliced onion, bell peppers, and tomato.
8. Drizzle the salad with olive oil, lemon juice, and salt and pepper.
9. Serve salad afterward.

Whole Cooked Cauliflower

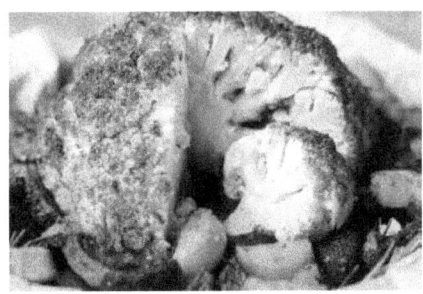

Preparation time: **15 minutes**
Cooking time: **5 hours**

Serve: 4

Ingredients:
- 1 large head cauliflower
- 2 cloves garlic, minced
- 3 tablespoons coconut oil, melted and cooled
- 3 tablespoons lemon juice
- 2 teaspoons lemon zest
- Salt and pepper, to taste
- 2 tablespoons chopped parsley
- 2 teaspoons coriander powder

Instructions:
1. Clean the cauliflower from any outer green leaves.
2. In a small bowl, combine garlic, coconut oil, coriander powder, and lemon juice.
3. Pour the mixture over cauliflower and rub it in gently.
4. Sprinkle the cauliflower with salt and pepper and place inside your slow cooker.
5. Pour lemon juice around the cauliflower and close the cooker with a lid.
6. Cook the cauliflower on low for 5 hours.
7. Serve the cauliflower warm.

Jacket Potatoes

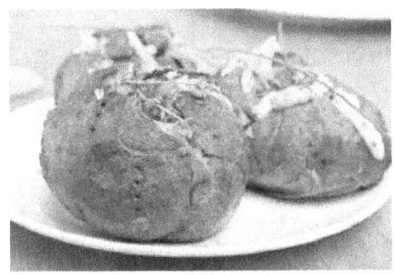

Preparation time: **10 minutes**
Cooking time: **4 hours**
Serve: 4

Ingredients:
- 4 baking potatoes
- 1 tablespoon olive oil
- Salt and pepper, to taste

Instructions:
- Wash and dry each potato.
- Prick potatoes with a toothpick or fork and brush with olive oil. Season each potato with salt and pepper and wrap in aluminum foil.
- Place the potatoes in a slow cooker and close with the lid. Cook the potatoes on low for 4 hours (if small) or 5 hours (if medium).

- Unwrap the potatoes and serve with desired toppings or as a side dish.

Slow Cooker Desserts

Tapioca Pudding

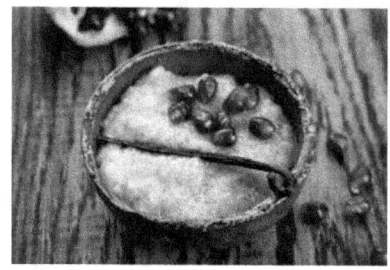

Preparation time: **10 minutes**
Cooking time: **6 hours**
Serve: 4

Ingredients:
- 3 cups almond milk
- ½ cup coconut sugar
- ½ cup tapioca pearls
- 1 vanilla bean, seeds scraped
- 1 small pinch salt
- Pomegranate seeds, to serve with

Instructions:
1. In a slow cooker, combine almond milk, coconut sugar, tapioca, vanilla seeds, and salt.

2. Stir gently and cook on low for 6-8 hours. This should be stirred a few times while cooking.
3. Serve pudding topped with pomegranate seeds.

Apple Crumble

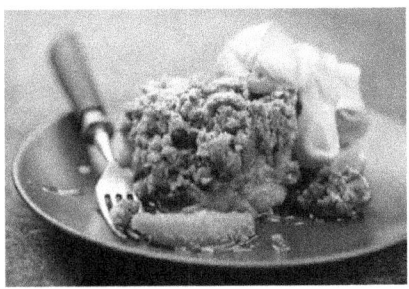

Preparation time: **10 minutes**
Cooking time: **8 hours**
Serve: 6

Ingredients:
- 6 apples, peeled, cored, and sliced
- 3 tablespoons maple syrup
- 1 teaspoon Ceylon cinnamon or plain cinnamon
- ¼ teaspoon nutmeg
- 2 tablespoons coconut oil, softened
- 3 cups Vegan granola*

Instructions:
1. Arrange the apples in a slow cooker.

2. Drizzle the apples with maple syrup.
3. Sprinkle the apples with cinnamon, nutmeg, and top with coconut oil.
4. Cover the apples with granola and bake on low for 8 hours.
5. Serve the apple crumble warm with some vanilla ice cream.

*NOTE: to make the Vegan granola, combine ½ cup rolled oats, ¾ cup chopped pecans, and 2 tablespoons maple syrup. Spread the mixture over the baking sheet, lined with baking paper. Bake the granola 30 minutes, stirring halfway through. Cool completely before use.

Chocolate Fondue

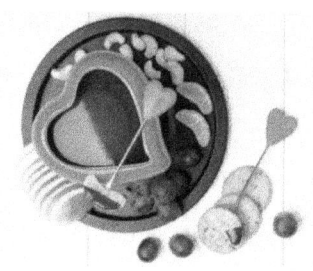

Preparation time: **5 minutes**
Cooking time: **1 hour**
Serve: 4

Ingredients:

- 1 cup dairy-free chocolate chips
- 4oz. 70% cacao-rich chocolate
- 1 cup coconut cream (from the can) *
- ½ cup almond milk
- 2 tablespoons cocoa butter
- 1 teaspoon vanilla paste or extract
- 1 pinch salt

Serve with:
- Sliced banana
- Sliced apples
- Strawberries
- Black grapes

Instructions:
1. Combine all the fondue ingredients in a slow cooker.
2. Cook on low for 1 hour.
3. Transfer the fondue in a serving bowl and serve with desired fruits.

*NOTE: you will get coconut cream if you place your can of full-fat coconut milk in a fridge overnight. Just open carefully in the morning and pick up the solids. Whip gently and use.

Slow Cooked Pudding

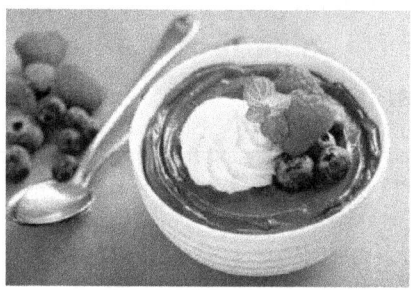

Preparation time: 10 minutes + inactive time
Cooking time: 1 hour 10 minutes
Serve: 4

Ingredients:
- 2 cups coconut milk
- 1 ¼ cup almond milk
- 3 tablespoons cacao powder or carob powder
- 4 tablespoons arrowroot starch or cornstarch
- 2/3 cup dairy-free chocolate chips
- 1 teaspoon vanilla paste
- 1 pinch salt

Serve with:
- Fresh berries
- Whipped coconut cream

Instructions:

1. Combine coconut milk, cacao powder, chocolate chips, and vanilla paste in a slow cooker.
2. Cover and cook on low for 40 minutes.
3. In the meantime, beat almond milk, salt, and arrowroot starch until smooth.
4. Whisk the arrowroot mixture into the slow cooker.
5. Continue to cook for 30 minutes on low.
6. Transfer the pudding into serving bowls.
7. Cover and refrigerate for 1 hour.
8. Serve topped with whipped cream and desired berries.

Carrot Cake

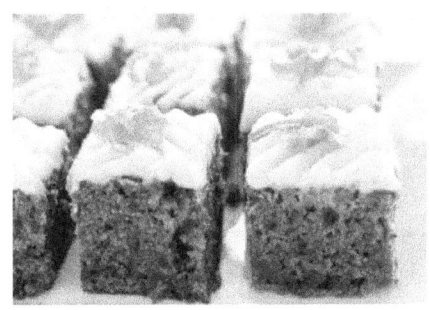

Preparation time: 15 minutes
Cooking time: 2 hours
Serve: 6

Ingredients:
- 1 cup all-purpose flour
- ¾ teaspoon baking powder

- ½ teaspoon baking soda
- 1 teaspoon ground cinnamon
- ¼ teaspoon ground nutmeg
- 2 small bananas, mashed
- ½ cup coconut sugar
- ¼ cup coconut oil
- 1 cup grated carrots
- 1/3 cup chopped pecans

Topping:
- ½ cup aquafaba (chickpea water from the can or collected when cooking chickpeas)
- 3 tablespoons coconut sugar

Instructions:
1. Make the cake; grease the slow cooker with some coconut oil.
2. Combine all-purpose flour, baking powder, baking soda, cinnamon, and nutmeg.
3. In a separate bowl, cream coconut oil with coconut sugar and banana.
4. Fold in the dry ingredients along with carrots and pecans.
5. Pour the batter in the slow cooker and smooth the top.
6. Cover and bake on low for 2 hours.
7. Turn off the slow cooker and let the cake rest for 30 minutes.
8. In the meantime, beat aquafaba with coconut sugar until whipped.

9. Remove the cake from the slow cooker. Top with whipped aquafaba.
10. Slice and serve.

Peached Peaches With Yogurt

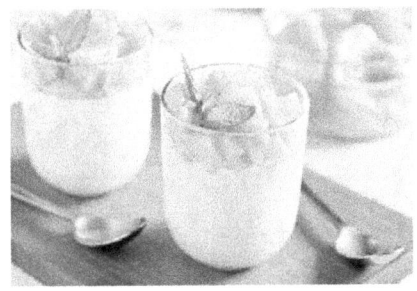

Preparation time: 10 minutes
Cooking time: 2 hours
Serve: 4

Ingredients
- 1lb. ripe peach pitted and thinly sliced
- 2 strips lemon zest
- 2 tablespoons maple syrup
- 1 pinch salt
- ½ cup hot water

Serve with:
- 2 cups almond yogurt
- 1 tablespoon toasted and chopped hazelnuts

Instructions:
1. Combine peaches, lemon zest, maple syrup, salt, and pour in water.
2. Cover and cook on low for 2 hours.
3. Let the peaches cool for 30 minutes.
4. Divide yogurt among four serving glasses. Sprinkle with almonds and top with peaches.
5. Serve.

Zebra Cake

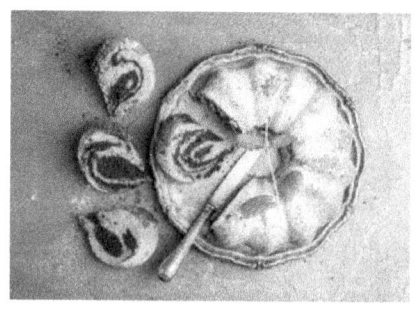

Preparation time: **15 minutes**
Cooking time: 2 hours 30 minutes
Serve: 6

Ingredients:
- 1 ½ cups all-purpose flour
- 1 cup coconut sugar
- 1 teaspoon baking soda
- 1 cup almond milk
- 2 tablespoons cacao powder
- 1/3 cup coconut oil
- 1 tablespoon lemon juice
- 1 teaspoon vanilla paste

Instructions:
1. Line bottom of your slow cooker with parchment paper.
2. In a large bowl, combine all-purpose flour, coconut sugar, baking soda, almond milk, coconut oil, and vanilla paste.
3. Stir until well blended. Pour 1/3 of the mixture into a separate bowl. Stir in cocoa powder.
4. Pour around ¼ cup of white batter into slow cooker.
5. Place on top 3 tablespoons chocolate batter. Do not stir and let the batter spread on its own.
6. Continue to add layers until you have used all the batter.
7. Cover the cooker with lid and cook the cake on low for 1 hour.
8. Carefully remove the slow cooker inner pot and rotate by 180 degrees, with the lid on. Continue to cook the cake on low for 1 ½ hour.

9. Remove the cake from the slow cooker and let it stand for 10 minutes.
10. You can dust the cake with powdered Erythritol before serving.

Lemon Poppy Seeds Cake

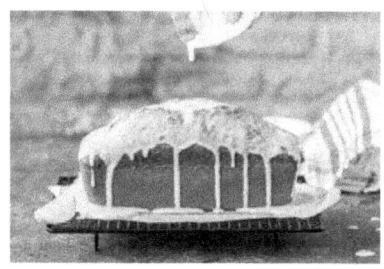

Preparation time: **15 minutes**
Cooking time: 2 hours 30 minutes
Serve: 8

Ingredients:
- 1 ½ cups all-purpose flour
- ½ cup coconut sugar
- 2 tablespoons poppy seeds
- ¾ teaspoon baking powder
- ¼ teaspoon baking soda
- 1 cup almond milk
- 1/3 cup coconut oil
- 1 ½ tablespoon lemon zest
- 3 tablespoons lemon juice

For the icing:
- ¾ cup powdered Erythritol
- 1 ½ tablespoon lemon juice

Instructions:
1. Line your cooker with parchment paper.
2. In a mixing bowl, combine flour, sugar, poppy seeds, baking powder, and baking soda.
3. In a separate bowl, beat almond milk, coconut oil, lemon zest, and lemon juice.
4. Fold the liquid ingredients into the dry ones.
5. Stir until smooth.
6. Pour the batter into the slow cooker.
7. Cover and cook on low for 2 ½ hours.
8. Let the cake rest for 10 minutes before removing from the slow cooker.
9. In the meantime, make the icing; whisk powdered Erythritol and lemon juice in a bowl.
10. Spread the icing over the cake.
11. Slice the cake and serve.

Lazy Berry Pie

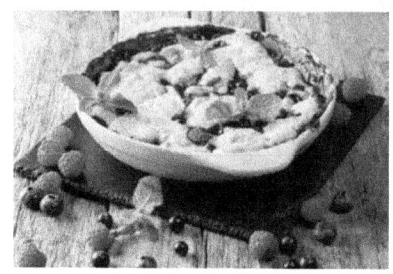

Preparation time: 10 minutes
Cooking time: 2 hours 30 minutes
Serve: 12

Ingredients:
- 1 ½ cups rolled oats, ground
- ½ cup whole-wheat flour
- ½ cup finely chopped almonds
- 2 tablespoons cornstarch
- 1/3 cup coconut oil
- 5 cups mixed berries
- 3 tablespoons maple syrup
- 2 teaspoons vanilla extract

Instructions:
1. Coat the slow cooker with cooking spray.

2. Combine oat, flour, 1 ½ tablespoon cornstarch, and almonds in a food blender. Add coconut oil and vanilla.
3. Process until you have coarse crumbs.
4. Toss the berries with remaining cornstarch and place into a slow cooker.
5. Top the berries with prepared flour mixture.
6. Cover and cook on low for 2 ½ hours.
7. Serve the crumble at room temperature.

Lemon Dessert

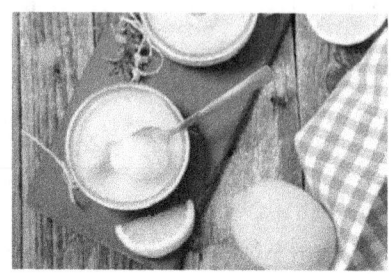

Preparation time: 5 minutes

Cooking time: 1 hour 30 minutes

Serve: 6

Ingredients:

- 14oz. can of low-fat coconut milk
- 2 tablespoons arrowroot starch
- ½ cup freshly squeezed lemon juice
- 2 tablespoons finely grated lemon zest
- 2 tablespoons maple syrup

Instructions:

1. Whisk all ingredients in a slow cooker.
2. Cover and cook on low for 1 ½ hour.
3. Remove the lid and whisk the custard before dividing among six serving bowls.
4. Refrigerate the custard for 1 hour before serving.

Conclusion

Being healthy and consuming delicious food at the same time couldn't get any easier than this. Every Vegan understands the importance of nutritional and tasty food. And once you're through reading this book, you won't have any difficulties in creating your own vegan slow cooker masterpieces within a matter of days!

We hope you have found your favorite recipe and realized cooking can be easy while being able to enjoy quality meals.

Part 2

Introduction To Vegan Slow Cooking

A slow cooker or crockpot is an electrical cooking appliance used for simmering and allows unattended cooking of a variety of dishes. There is a lot to be said for a device that does the cooking for you while you are sleeping or away at work or busy doing something else around the house and greets you with appetizing aromas and fragrances upon your return. For many vegans, slow cookers hold little or no significance as people have typically come to associate them with tough cuts of meat or hearty roasts. That's where they are mistaken! Whether it is savory soups or juicy stews, crock pots can do it all and much more and this article will aim to elaborate on how you can use your slow cooker for vegan recipes.

Although the slow cooker may, at one time, have been synonymous with cooking meat dishes and steaks, there are a wide variety of vegan dishes that can be made with this versatile appliance and we are not just talking about the usual fare of soups and stews; there are recipes for chilis, risottos, casseroles, sauces, breads and even a number of desserts -- all vegan and all that can be made in the slow cooker! The best part is the flavor of any dish produced from this cooking appliance; the slow, stewing process allows all the different flavors to merge and absorb, augmenting the taste of the dish tenfold. This is a cooking process that cannot be compared to any other.

Slow cookers are also extremely simple to use, all you need to do is plug it in and pour in the ingredients -- the rest will all be done by the device itself. It's almost like having your own personal chef! It is not only convenient but the dishes it produces are nothing to complain about either. The slow process brings out more flavor and nutrients from the ingredients producing food that not only tastes better but is also healthier. For many vegans, slow cookers are the epitome of a healthier, more convenient and more economical lifestyle.

Although many vegan dishes just require you to deposit the ingredients and wait, other may require a few additional processes such as stir frying vegetables before putting them into the slow cooker to produce a better final result. Compared to meat recipes in the crock pot, vegan recipes also cook faster. If you are a vegan looking for delicious recipes that can be made at your convenience, then slow cooking is definitely the answer for you.

Benefits of Veganism

Veganism is more of a lifestyle choice and a philosophy than just a different kind of diet. Vegan diets include only plant-based foods, and the exclusion of all products of animal origin. There are a few specific reasons people adopt this kind of diet; these are usually related to the environment, health or animal rights. Most vegans believe in the freedom of animals- to exist without interference from human beings. Others believe that livestock farming is inefficient and promotes environmental damage such as top soil erosion, water pollution etc. However, for many, the most important reason for veganism is also a significant benefit arising from it i.e. good health.

Lower chances of illnesses: Animal fats mostly consist of cholesterol, fats and proteins and can increase a person's chance of developing cancer, diabetes, heart disease and hypertension. Foods like vegetables, whole grain and legumes do not contain cholesterol and have low fat content, especially saturated fats. They are also high in fiber, healthy proteins and many other nutrients. A cardio-protective diet, paired with the heavy emphasis vegans place on fruits and vegetables, results in a high potassium regime which is associated with the moderation of blood pressure. A vegan diet can also help regulate blood sugar, naturally.

Improved digestion/ Energy levels: Veganism contributes towards improved digestion: with all that fiber added to your diet- it makes sure to keep things going the way they are supposed to. It is also said to have a positive impact upon energy levels; most vegans talk about how much unexpected energy they suddenly seem to have soon after switching to this diet.

Weight Loss/ Maintenance: A vegan regime can help you lose weight to your desired target and more importantly, to keep it there! Since vegan foods are typically lower in calories and unhealthy fats, this makes it easier for vegans to maintain a healthy weight. For people who are over-weight or even those who just have trouble regulating their weight at a certain level this is a great diet to do both.

Benefits for the Environment:The benefits of a vegan diet extend beyond our own health and include a positive impact on the environment as well. A plant-based diet dramatically reduces a number of issues. It allows more efficient use to be made of land and water, protects forests (to be used as grazing land) from destruction and also promotes less pollution.

Benefits for Animals: Concern for the way farm animals are treated and objections to the use and slaughter of animals is another reason to go vegan. Humans don't need animal products to feed or clothe themselves and with an increasing awareness of the cramped, filthy conditions in many factory farms, choosing a vegan diet becomes an even easier choice, reflecting compassion for these animals on a daily basis.

You've made a great decision in deciding on a Vegan lifestyle. The following recipes are delicious, healthy, and easy to make for busy professionals. Now onto the recipes!

Chilis, Soups, And Stews

Rich Mushroom And Tortellini Soup With White Sauce

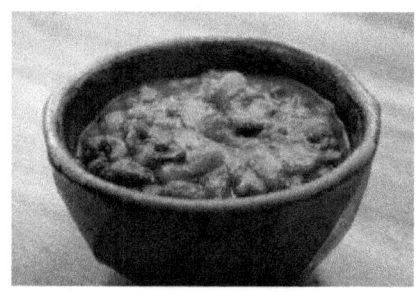

Description: Creamy white sauce, soft luscious mushrooms and a sprinkling of parmesan result in a rich soup- both pleasant and refreshing. Add the mouth watering aroma of oregano, stir in some fresh spinach and eat with bread on the side for a satisfyingly delightful meal.

Ingredients:
- 1 envelope white sauce mix (1 ½- 2 oz.)
- 4 cups water
- 1 can vegetable broth (14 oz.)
- 1 ½ cups fresh mushrooms, sliced
- ½ cup onion, chopped
- 3 cloves garlic, minced

- ½ teaspoonful dried basil, crushed
- ¼ teaspoonful salt
- ¼ teaspoonful dried oregano, crushed
- 1/8 teaspoonful cayenne pepper
- 1 7 - 8 oz. package dried cheese tortellini (about 2 cups)
- 1 can evaporated milk (12 oz.)
- 6 cups fresh baby spinach leaves or torn spinach
- Ground black pepper (optional)
- Finely shredded Parmesan cheese (optional)

Directions:

Use a 3 ½ or 4 quart slow cooker; add the white sauce mix and gradually start stirring in water until smooth. Add the broth, onion, basil, cayenne pepper, oregano, salt, garlic and mushrooms to the white sauce. Cover and let the ingredients cook on a low setting for 5 ½ hours or a high setting for 3 hours. Mix in the tortellini and cook again on a low setting for an hour or on a high setting for 45 minutes.

Finally, add the evaporated milk and the fresh spinach. You may sprinkle black pepper and Parmesan cheese on individual servings. This recipe makes four servings.

Red Bean Noodle Soup

Description: Herb-infused, hot and spicy soup with a delicious combination of beans and noodles. Makes a rewarding meal, garnished with fresh parsley and grated cheese and paired with some warm, crusty bread.

Ingredients:

- 1 cup cooked kidney beans, drained & rinsed
- 1 cup dry spaghetti, cooked al dente, rinsed with cold water, and set aside
- 1 tablespoonful olive oil
- 1 tablespoonful minced fresh garlic (2 - 3 cloves)
- ¼ cup diced onion
- 1 minced fresh jalapeño pepper
- 1 medium carrot, peeled and sliced thin on the diagonal
- 2 stalks celery, trimmed and sliced thinly
- 1 medium potato, peeled and cut in 1" cubes
- 1 cup sliced fresh or frozen green beans
- ½ chopped red bell pepper
- 1/8 teaspoonful cayenne or chipotle pepper
- 1 teaspoonful dried basil
- ½ teaspoonful dried oregano leaf
- ½ teaspoonful dried thyme leaf
- 1 tsp dried marjoram leaf
- ½ teaspoonful ground cumin
- 1 teaspoonful ground coriander
- 1 cup low sodium tomato sauce
- ½ teaspoonful salt or to taste
- 4 cups water or soup stock
- ¼ cup chopped fresh basil, parsley or cilantro as garnish

- Optional: grated dairy or non-dairy cheese

Directions:

Boil water and cook spaghetti for approximately 7 minutes before rinsing with cold water and setting aside.

In a pan, heat oil and add onions. Fry for 5 minutes on medium heat before adding garlic and jalapeño; sauté for another 5 minutes and then add celery, carrot, potato, red pepper, green beans and herbs and spices; sauté for approximately 5 to 7 minutes further. Drain and rinse the kidney beans and add to the vegetables with water/stock and tomato sauce.

Add all the ingredients to a slow cooker excluding the spaghetti and frozen beans. Put on the lid and cook on a low setting for 4 to 6 hours or until vegetables are tender. Add pasta, frozen beans and salt. Turn on high setting and simmer for approximately 20 minutes. Serve with fresh herbs and grated cheese!

Greek Vegetable Stew With Feta Cheese

Description: A twist on the usual version of stew; this recipe combines vegetables with exquisite spices to add just the right amount of flavor. Serve with hot couscous and feta cheese to make it stand out! You can even replace the vegetables with other ones of your own preference.

Ingredients:

- 2 cups butternut squash, cubed
- 2 cups carrots, chopped
- 2 onions, chopped
- 1 cup zucchini, chopped
- 2 cans diced tomatoes, undrained (14 oz. cans)
- 15 oz. can garbanzo beans, rinsed and drained
- 14 oz. can vegetable broth
- 2 cloves garlic, minced
- 1 tsp. cumin
- 1/2 tsp. salt
- 1/2 tsp. allspice
- 1/4 tsp. pepper
- 1/2 tsp. ground coriander
- 4 cups hot, cooked couscous
- 1/2 cup crumbled feta cheese

Directions:

In a 3 to 4 quart slow cooker, add all the vegetables, the broth, garlic, cumin, salt, allspice, pepper and coriander. Stir to combine well and then cook (covered) on a low setting for 7 to 9 hours or until veggies becomes tender. Serve with hot couscous and a sprinkling of feta cheese. This recipe makes 6 servings.

Spicy Vegan Chili

Description: For some, chili without beef is unthinkable but this recipe is enough to convince any disbelievers. All the ingredients, merged together, form an out-of-this-world texture; the fiery flavor will entice your taste buds and have you asking for more. If you're looking for an appetizing, mind-numbingly awesome chili recipe, you've got yourself a winner!

Ingredients:

- 4 cups black beans
- 2 teaspoonfuls cumin
- 3 tablespoonfuls chili powder
- 4 cups tomatoes (diced), with juice
- 1 onion, chopped
- 1 teaspoonful salt
- 1 teaspoonful black pepper
- 1 teaspoonful garlic powder
- 2 cups ground lentil and rice beef substitute
- 1 green pepper, chopped
- 1 teaspoonful chipotle pepper seasoning (optional, to add extra spice)

Directions:

Add, pepper, garlic powder, chili powder, cumin and chipotle pepper to a bowl and mix all the spices together. Grease a 4-quart slow cooker and add all the ingredients, followed by the spice mixture. Cook for 8 to 10 hours on low setting or 4 to 6 hours on high. Serve while it's hot!

Divine Tomato And Chickpea Soup

Description: This deliciously creamy tomato soup is full of flavor with a perfect, thick texture to satisfy even the most avid soup lover. Seasoned with fresh herbs or parmesan cheese, it offers an amazing blend of flavors and aroma; an excellent choice for a cold, winter evening.

Ingredients:

- 2 cans chickpeas, drained & rinsed (16 oz. cans)
- 4 cups water or bean broth
- 2 vegetable bouillon cubes, unsalted
- 6 ripe plum tomatoes OR 1 large can crushed unsalted tomatoes
- 2 bay leaves
- 1 tablespoonful raw cane or turbinado sugar
- 2 tablespoonfuls olive oil
- 2 large carrots, chopped
- 2 celery stalks, diced
- 2 cloves garlic (peeled, cored and minced)
- 1 teaspoonful cumin
- 1 teaspoonful smoked paprika
- 1 pinch chipotle pepper or to taste

- 1 tablespoonful dried basil, or ½ fresh basil chopped
- ½ teaspoon salt
- 1 tablespoonful Braggs liquid aminos or low sodium soy sauce
- 2 tablespoonfuls tomato paste
- 2 tablespoonfuls minced fresh parsley or basil

Directions:

Boil the cooked and drained chickpeas in a sauce pan with water, vegetable cubes and bay leaves. Cover the saucepan and let it simmer.

Heat oil in a pot, add the minced garlic and fry for two minutes. Then add the chopped carrots and celery and stir fry. Add cumin, paprika, chipotle pepper and basil and keep stirring. After two minutes, turn the heat up and add the tomatoes, stir fry them for five minutes. Add the chickpeas and stock mixture and bring to a boil.

Pour the boiled mixture into a slow cooker and allow it to cook on low heat for 4 hours. Add tomato paste, salt, pepper and Braggs liquid and mix it all in. Blend soup with a blender stick and season with shredded mozzarella, parmesan or fresh herbs. Serve warm.

Potatoes And Dumplings

Cheesy Potatoes Au Gratin In The Slow Cooker

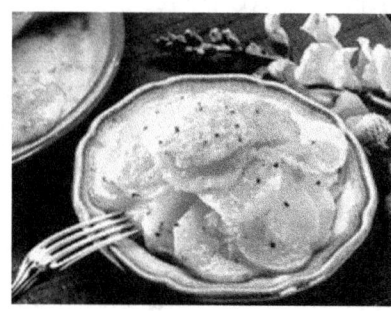

Description: An effortless recipe that tastes like heaven; the thinly sliced potatoes layered with cheese that melts in your mouth provide the perfect excuse to cheat on your diet. Add some French fried onion straws to the side to make them taste even better!

Ingredients:
- 2-3 Potatoes, thinly sliced
- Sliced Onion (Optional)
- 2 Cups Soy Milk
- 1 Cup Daiya Vegan Cheddar Shreds
- 2 tablespoonfuls Whole Wheat Flour
    - **Pepper**
- French Fried Onion Straws (Optional)

Directions:

In a bowl, add the whole wheat flour, soy milk and some pepper to taste; whisk together until well combined.

Layer the sliced potatoes into your crock pot, followed by a layer of sliced onions and cheese. Keep adding as many layers as you want. Pour the flour mixture on top and cover the slow cooker. Cook on a low setting for 7 hours or a high setting for 4 to 5 hours or until potatoes are tender. Serve with French fried onion straws!

Dumplings With Stewed Veggies

Description: Cornmeal dumplings paired with a succulent vegetable stew and a hint of Parmesan cheese and parsley; this is a delightful vegan dish with an Italian flair.

Ingredients:
- 3 cups peeled butternut or acorn squash cut into 1/2-inch cubes
- 2 cups fresh mushrooms, julienned
- 2 cans diced tomatoes, undrained (14 ½ oz. cans)
- 1 can beans, rinsed and drained (15 oz.)
- 1 cup water
- 4 cloves garlic, minced
- 1 teaspoonful dried Italian seasoning, crushed
- ¼ teaspoonful ground black pepper
- ½ cup all-purpose flour
- 1/3 cup cornmeal

- 2 tablespoonfuls grated Parmesan cheese
- 1 tablespoonful snipped fresh parsley
- 1 teaspoonful baking powder
- ¼ teaspoonful salt
- **1 egg**
- 2 tablespoonfuls milk
- 2 tablespoonfuls cooking oil
- 1 package frozen Italian green beans or frozen cut green beans (9 oz.)
- **Paprika**

Directions:

For Dumplings

Combine flour, cornmeal, parsley, Parmesan cheese, salt and baking powder in a bowl and mix together well. In another bowl, add milk, oil and egg and beat. Add the liquid mixture to the flour mixture and beat with a fork until well combined.

For Vegetable Stew

Use a 3 ½ or 4 quart crock pot. Add the mushrooms, tomatoes, squash, beans, water garlic, pepper and Italian seasoning. Cover the cooker and cook for approximately 9 hours on a low setting or 4 ½ hours on a high setting.

If using low setting, turn to high setting and stir frozen beans into the stew. Pour in the dumpling batter in six equal portions on top of the stew and sprinkle with paprika. Cook for 50 minutes more and make sure the lid is not lifted while dumplings are cooking. This recipe makes 6 servings.

Savory Pies And Casseroles

Cheesy Tortellini Casserole With Tomato Sauce

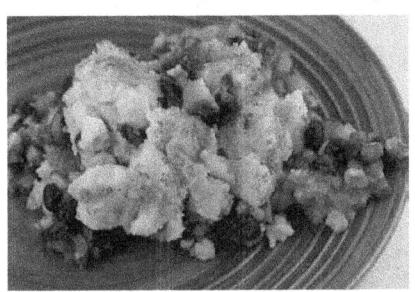

Description: A super-easy meatless recipe that will have you wanting more! This dish is tempting to look at, mouthwateringly delicious to eat and has an aroma that will draw you towards it immediately. Ravioli with chopped onions in a mild, garlicky tomato sauce, topped with a wonderful cheesy flavor makes for a splendid dish with an unbelievably short preparation time.

Ingredients:
- 3 cloves garlic, minced
- 1 onion, chopped
- 1 can or jar of spaghetti sauce (26 oz.)
- 1 can tomato sauce (8 oz.)
- 2 packages refrigerated ravioli or tortellini (9 oz. packages)
- 2 cups mozzarella cheese, shredded

Directions:

Use a 4 to 6 quart slow cooker. Add the chopped onion and garlic with spaghetti sauce and tomato sauce and mix well, stirring all the ingredients together. Put on the lid and simmer on a low setting for 8 to 9 hours or until onion appears to be tender. Add the tortellini and turn the setting on high. Cook for an hour. Sprinkle with cheese and cook 5 minutes longer to let the cheese melt. This recipe serves 8.

Crock Pot Shepherd's Pie

Ingredients:
- 1 (15-ounce) can black beans, drained and rinsed
- 1 (15-ounce) can kidney beans, drained and rinsed
- 1 (16-ounce) package frozen corn
- 1 small onion, diced
- 1 (15-ounce) can tomato sauce
- 1 teaspoon ground cumin
- 1/2 teaspoon kosher salt
- 1/2 teaspoon black pepper
- 1 cup shredded cheddar cheese
- 2 cups mashed potatoes (leftover, fresh, from a box-- your choice!)
- 1/2 teaspoon smoked paprika
-

Directions:

Use a 4-quart slow cooker. Drain and rinse the beans, and add to the crockpot. Add corn and diced onion.

Pour in the tomato sauce, and add cumin, salt, pepper. Stir well to combine. Sprinkle the shredded cheese evenly over the top.

Squish the 2 cups of mashed potatoes down on your chili with the back of a wooden spoon. Now dust with the smoked paprika.

Cover and cook on low for 5-6 hours, or on high for 3-4. Uncover the slow cooker near serving time and let cook uncovered on high for 20-30 minutes to cook away any collected condensation. The potatoes will brown on top a tiny bit and begin to pull from the sides.

Cheesy Slow Cooker Casserole

Description: A different kind of vegan casserole infused with colorful herbs, spices and cheese. A mixture of juicy and crunchy vegetables exploding with the flavor of basil pesto, garlic and Italian seasoning, make this one recipe you definitely want to give a try!

Ingredients:
- 2 can cannellini beans (19 oz. cans)
- 1 can garbanzo or fava beans (19 oz.)
- ¼ cup purchased basil pesto
- 1 medium onion, chopped
- 4 cloves garlic, minced
- 1 ½ teaspoons dried Italian seasoning, crushed
- 1 package refrigerated cooked plain polenta cut in 1/2-inch-thick slices (16 oz.)
- 1 large tomato, thinly sliced

- 2 cups finely shredded Italian cheese blend (8 oz.)
- 2 cups fresh spinach
- 1 cup torn radicchio

Directions:

Rinse beans and drain and add them to a large bowl with 2 tablespoons of pesto, onion, garlic and Italian seasoning.

In a 4 to 5 quart crock pot, layer the bottom with half of the bean mixture, half of the polenta and half of the cheese. Add the remaining beans and polenta. Put on the lid and cook on a low setting for 4 to 6 hours or on a high setting for 2 to 2 ½ hours. Add tomato, the remaining cheese, spinach and radicchio. Combine the remaining pesto with 1 tablespoon of water and sprinkle it over the casserole.

This recipe makes 8 servings.

Creamy Vegetable Pie

Description: This tasty pie pairs soft, warm vegetables, cooked in a buttery sauce, with a crisp and crunchy biscuit topping to produce the perfect combination of flavors and textures. From the moment you smell the delicious aroma of this mouth watering dish, you won't be able to stay away.

Ingredients:

For the filling:

- 2 tablespoonfuls olive oil or non-dairy margarine
- 2 cups baking potato, diced and peeled

- 2 cups carrot, diced
- 1 cup celery, chopped
- ½ teaspoonful salt
- ½ teaspoonful freshly ground black pepper
- 2 garlic cloves, minced
- 2 ½ tablespoonfuls whole wheat pastry flour
- 1 ½ cup organic or non-dairy milk (unflavored and unsweetened)
- ¾ cup vegetable broth
- 2 cups frozen green peas
- 1 can of chickpeas, drained and rinsed (14 ½ oz.)
- 1 teaspoonful dried thyme
- 1 teaspoonful dried basil
- ½ teaspoonful dried oregano

For the biscuit topping:

- 1 cup organic or non-dairy milk (unflavored and unsweetened)
- 2 teaspoonfuls lemon juice or apple cider vinegar
- 1 1/3 cup whole wheat pastry flour
- 1/3 cup unbleached all purpose flour
- 1 ½ teaspoonfuls baking powder
- ¾ teaspoonfuls baking soda
- ¼ teaspoonfuls salt
- ½ teaspoonfuls freshly ground black pepper
- 4 ½ tablespoonfuls non-dairy margarine, cut into pieces
- 1/3 cup grated fresh Parmesan cheese or nutritional yeast

- ½ teaspoonfuls dried basil

Directions:

For the filling:

Heat a large pan on medium heat and add 1 ½ teaspoons of non-dairy margarine, followed by potatoes, carrots, celery, salt and pepper. Sauté all the ingredients for approximately 5 minutes, making sure the vegetables become tender. Then add garlic and sauté for a couple of minutes, allowing the garlic flavor to merge with the other ingredients.

In a separate pan, add the remaining 1 ½ tablespoons of margarine and 2 ½ tablespoons flour and whisk for one minute. Gradually add milk and both while whisking slowly and cook until the sauce starts getting thick.

In a 5 quart crock, add the sautéed vegetables and the sauce. Start stirring in the peas, chickpeas, thyme, basil and oregano and season with salt and pepper. Cook for about 3 ½ hours , allowing vegetables to become tender.

For the biscuit topping:

Combine milk and lemon juice in a bowl and set it aside. To another bowl, add flour, baking powder, baking soda, salt and pepper and then start cutting in butter until the texture of the mixture becomes course. Stir in cheese and the soured milk until mixture is moist.

Final Step:

Increase the slow cooker setting to high and spoon in the biscuit topping in eight equal portions. Cook on high for 1 hour and 15 minutes. When your pie is done, uncover it and let it cool for five to ten minutes before serving. This recipe serves 6.

Easy Crock Pot Veggie-Loaf

Description: A meal that cooks itself (pretty much!) and smells and tastes delicious; what's not to like? The mouthwatering aroma of this vegan meatloaf will draw you towards it from afar and the distinctive, delightful taste will have you begging for more. A satisfying and healthy dish for lunch or dinner; it's a dream come true for any vegan foodie out there.

Ingredients:
- 2 teaspoonfuls olive oil, plus more for drizzling
- 1 small yellow onion, minced
- 2 garlic cloves, minced
- 1 tablespoonful dried thyme
- 1 can beans, rinsed and drained (15 oz. can)
- 12 oz. extra-firm tofu, drained, squeezed, and crumbled
- ¾ cup ketchup
- 2 tablespoonfuls vegan Worcestershire sauce or soy sauce
- 1 tablespoonful Dijon mustard
- ½ cup ground walnuts
- ½ cup old-fashioned rolled oats

- ¼ cup dried bread crumbs
- ½ cup vital wheat gluten
- Gluten Free Option: ½ cup chick pea flour or potato flour
- 2 tablespoonfuls tapioca starch
- 2 tablespoonfuls minced fresh flat-leaf parsley
- Salt and freshly ground black pepper
- 2 large carrots, peeled and cut into ¼-inch slices
- 2 or 3 Yukon Gold potatoes, peeled and cut into ½-inch slices
- 2 or 3 shallots, quartered lengthwise
- 2 tablespoonfuls yellow or brown mustard
- 1 tablespoonful light brown sugar
- 1 tablespoonful cider vinegar

Directions:

In a small skillet, heat 2 teaspoons of oil and stir fry the onions for about five minutes, until light brown and soft. Add garlic and thyme and cook for 2 minutes. Set this mixture aside.

Combine beans, tofu, ½ cup of ketchup, Worcestershire, mustard and the onion mixture in a food processor and process until the ingredients are combined well.

Add walnuts, oats, wheat gluten, tapioca starch, bread crumbs and parsley to a large bowl and mix together. Season the mixture with a teaspoon of salt and ¼ teaspoon of black pepper. Add the processed bean mixture to the bowl and stir thoroughly. Turn it out onto a wok surface and shape into an oval or round shape in order to fit it inside your crock pot. Keep pressing to ensure the load holds well together.

Grease the inside of a 5 to 7 quart slow cooker and arrange the carrot slices at the bottom. Season with salt and pepper and then layer the carrot slices with potato slices. Sprinkle some olive oil and set the rounded loaf on top of the potatoes, surrounding it with shallots.

Add the remaining ketchup to a small bowl with mustard, brown sugar and vinegar and stir thoroughly. Spread the mixture on top of the loaf in the slow cooker. Cook on a low setting for 4 hours. Once it is cooked, remove the lid and allow the loaf to cool for 10 to 15 minutes before carefully transferring it onto a serving platter. Surround with carrots, potatoes and shallots and your veggie-loaf is ready to eat.

Pasta, Noodles, And Rice

Vegan Mushroom And Spinach Lasagna

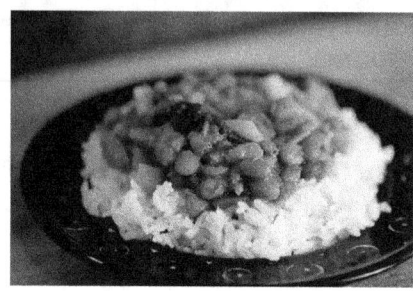

Description: An all-in-one lasagna with mushrooms and spinach in a light tomato garlic sauce and the classic flavor of Italian seasoning; this dish is absolutely irresistible!

Ingredients:
- 2 cups tomato sauce
- 4-5 lasagna noodles
- 1 cup frozen mushrooms, sliced
- 1 ½ cups frozen chopped spinach
- 2 cups vegan burger crumbles
- 2 tablespoons minced garlic
- 2 tablespoons Italian seasoning

Directions:

Layer the bottom of your slow cooker with a small amount of tomato sauce; just enough to cover the base. Break the lasagna noodles into pieces that will fit inside the crock pot and place them on top the layer of tomato sauce. Sprinkle one tablespoon of the sauce over the noodles and add mushrooms. Proceed by adding another layer of noodles over the mushrooms; sprinkle a tablespoon of sauce and half of the spinach. Add a third layer of noodles plus one cup of the burger crumbles. Scatter the minced garlic and Italian seasoning. Continue layering until all the ingredients are finished.

Cook on a low setting for 4 to 5 hours. Serve with some heated tomato sauce on the side and a sprinkling of cheese.

Tofu Teriyaki With Steamed Rice

Description: Crusty tofu swimming in delicious gravy that's a cross between barbecue and teriyaki, served with hot steamed rice, makes for a great addition to any dinner or lunch menu. Add some steamed vegetables to the side to add a nice, colorful touch to the final presentation.

Ingredients:
- ½ white onion
- 1 package of extra firm tofu
- ½ cup gluten free teriyaki sauce
- 2 tablespoonfuls white wine vinegar
- 1 tablespoonful Worcestershire sauce
- 1 teaspoonful cinnamon
- ½ teaspoonful fennel
- ½ teaspoonful ginger

- ½ teaspoonful cloves
- ½ teaspoonful red pepper flakes

Directions:

Drain and put some weight on the tofu to get rid of the extra moisture. You can do this procedure over night as well. Cut into small, one inch cubes and stir fry in olive oil until it appears to be a nice golden brown on all sides.

Chop up your onion and add to your slow cooker, along with the teriyaki sauce, wine vinegar, Worcestershire sauce, cinnamon, fennel, ginger, cloves and red pepper. Toss in the tofu to coat it thoroughly. Put on the lid and cook on a low setting for 6 hours. Serve with steamed rice and vegetables.

Artichoke And Tomato Fettucine

Description: Herb-infused tomatoes tango with garlic, artichokes, and cream, creating a delightful pasta dish with Mediterranean flair.s

Ingredients:
- Nonstick cooking spray
- 3 cans diced tomatoes with basil, oregano, and garlic (14 ½ oz. cans)
- 2 cans artichoke hearts, drained and quartered (14 oz. cans)
- 6 cloves garlic, minced
- ½ cup whipping cream
- 12 oz. dried fettucine

- Sliced pimiento-stuffed green olives and/or sliced pitted ripe olives (optional)
- Crumbled feta cheese or finely shredded Parmesan cheese (optional)

Directions:

Use a 3 ½ or 4 quart crock pot and grease the inside with cooking spray. Drain two cans of tomatoes and leave the remaining one undrained. Add all the tomatoes (drained and undrained), artichoke hearts and garlic to the cooker and combine. Put on the lid and cook on a low setting for 6 to 7 hours or on a high setting for 3 to 4 hours. When cooked, stir in the whipping cream and let it stand for five minutes.

Cook the fettucine according to package directions and drain. Serve the cooked sauce over hot fettucine and top with olives and cheese. This recipe makes 6 servings.

Tofu Peanut Surprise With Rice

Ingredients:
- small package of extra-firm tofu (half of a double-pack)
- 1/2 cup natural peanut butter
- 2 T soy sauce (La Choy is gluten free, as is Tamari wheat-free)

- 3 T Margarita Mix (be quiet. we were out of limes. it worked!)
- 1/2 teaspoon ginger
- 2-3 cloves of chopped garlic (we're still out, so I had to use the jarred stuff)
- 1/4 teaspoon crushed red pepper flakes
- Whole bag of baby spinach

Directions:

Use a 2-4 quart crockpot for best results. Although I despise pre-cooking things before cooking in the crockpot, tofu is best when lightly browned. I've found the best way is to cube it, then toss with a tablespoon or so of cornstarch. Pan-fry on the stove in butter.

Add to crockpot with peanut butter, soy sauce, margarita mix, garlic and pepper flakes. Cover and cook on low for 3-4 hours. 15 minutes before serving, cram an entire bag of baby spinach inside and cover. The spinach will wilt. Serve over basmati rice.

Spicy Garbanzo Bean Curry With Brown Rice

Description: Each bite of this curry will produce a burst of flavor in your mouth; well-cooked garbanzo beans seasoned with an alluring and colorful array of spices- cumin, turmeric, chili powder and cayenne pepper. Eat with brown rice and add a dollop of Greek yogurt for fun.

Ingredients:

- 1 ½ cups dried black garbanzo beans
- 1 small onion, coarsely chopped
- ½ cup fresh tomato, chopped
- 2 teaspoonfuls minced ginger root
- 2 teaspoonfuls minced garlic
- ½ - 1 teaspoonful cayenne pepper
- 1 ½ teaspoonful cumin seeds
- ½ teaspoonful turmeric
- ½ teaspoonful chili powder
- 2 teaspoonful salt (or less)
- 1 can petite diced tomatoes (optional)
- ½ cup thinly sliced green onions (optional)
- 3-4 tablespoonfuls chopped fresh cilantro
- 1 tablespoonful fresh squeezed lemon juice
- Cooked brown rice

Directions:

Blend together the onion, tomatoes, ginger, garlic, cayenne, cumin seeds, turmeric, chili powder and salt in a food processor to make a puree. Put the beans in a 3 ½ quart slow cooker with 4 cups of water, add the puree and cook on a high setting for 9 hours or until beans become soft. It's a good idea to start checking on the beans after 6 hours and add more water if necessary.

Taste the curry and if it's not too spicy for your tastes there's no need to follow the additional steps. If it is; add the diced tomatoes and green onions and cook for another hour on a high setting.

In the end, mix in the chopped cilantro and lemon juice. Serve hot, over cooked brown rice.

Spicy Tofu-Broccoli Rice

Description: A healthy dish with a short preparation time-this rice recipe will become a regular feature on your menu. The different textures of tofu and spice coupled with brown rice and seasoned with some cayenne pepper and red chili powder to add a spicy flavor, make this an absolutely irresistible dish!

Ingredients:
- 1 ½ cups brown rice, I use medium grain
- 3 ¼ cups vegetable broth
- ½ cup nutritional yeast
- 1 lb broccoli floret
- 1 carton tofu (300 g)
- 1 teaspoonful red chili powder
- ¼ teaspoonful cayenne pepper (optional, for extra spice)

Directions:

Rinse rice and soak in water for at least an hour to improve the texture. Drain it and add it to a slow cooker, along with broth and yeast. Cook on a high setting for 1 ½ hours and then mix in the broccoli, tofu, chili powder and cayenne pepper. Add some more broth too if the mixture seems too dry. Cook for another 40 minutes, but keep checking every 15 minutes to see if broccoli is done.

Delectable Polenta And Kale Lasagna With Cheese Sauce

Description: Scrumptious lasagna that is both healthy and heavenly; what more could you ask for?! The tempting cheese sauce combined with the exotic zest of garlic and tanginess of marinara sauce make this dish a superb blend of flavors that you would not want to miss out on.

Ingredients:

For Lasagna
- 2 tablespoons olive oil
- Pre-made polenta slices
- 1 large portobello mushroom, cut into thin slices
- ½ bunch of kale, washed and chopped
- ½ large onion, finely chopped
- 4 cloves of garlic, minced
- 1 teaspoon dried basil
- Cheese sauce (see below)
- Salt and pepper to taste
- 1-2 cups marinara sauce

For Cheese Sauce
- 1 cup unsweetened non-dairy milk
- 1/3 cup raw cashews
- ¼ cup nutritional yeast
- 2 tablespoons soy sauce

- 1 tablespoon lemon juice
- 2 teaspoons Dijon mustard
- ½ teaspoon onion powder
- ½ teaspoon garlic powder
- 2 teaspoons corn starch or arrowroot
- ½ teaspoon white pepper

Directions:

For Cheese Sauce

Add all ingredients to a blender and blend until smooth.

For Lasagna

In a large cooking pot, heat 2 tablespoons of olive oil on medium heat. Add the sliced mushrooms and onions and stir fry until mushrooms start becoming juicy. Then add garlic and kale and cook until the kale starts to change color (becomes bright green) and softens. Pour in the cheese sauce and cook mixture until it starts to thicken. Taste and add salt and pepper, if necessary.

In the slow cooker, lay out a bottom layer of marinara sauce, then cover it with a single layer of polenta slices, followed by a layer of the mixture you cooked. Keep repeating this process and finish off with a layer of polenta and a final layer of marinara. Cook on a high heat setting for 3 to 4 hours. Let it cool for about 30 minutes before serving.

Mushroom Bouillon Stroganoff With Tempeh

Description: Juicy mushrooms, combined with bouillon and seasoned with tempeh make this recipe a delightful addition to any dinner menu. It's easy to prepare and tastes heavenly; savory and scrumptious- an excellent choice for a satiating meal.

Ingredients:
- 1 package (8 oz. or 227g) tempeh, chopped
- 2 cups mushrooms, chopped small
- 2 cloves garlic, minced
- 1 to 2 cups water
- 1 teaspoonful Not-Chicken Bouillon
- ½ teaspoonful paprika
- 1/3 cup vegan sour cream (sub cashew cream or unsweetened non-dairy milk)
- pinch dill, optional
- salt and pepper, to taste
- cooked pasta, for serving

Directions:

Steam tempeh for approximately 10 minutes to get rid of the bitter taste. Add the steamed tempeh, mushrooms, bouillon, garlic, water and paprika to a 1 ½ to 2 quart slow cooker and cook on a low setting for 8 hours. Season with salt and pepper and add more paprika according to your taste.

Mix in vegan sour cream before serving. Serve over boiled pasta and sprinkle with dill. Serves 2 to 3 persons.

Rice With Red Beans- New Orleans Style

Description: Appetizing to eat and simple to cook; a recipe to produce a delightfully enjoyable meal! Red beans simmer with celery and bell peppers, with an extra boost of flavor from garlic and Creole seasoning. Garnish with fresh mint leaves or chopped green onions to give it a unique touch.

Ingredients:
- 1 lb. dried red beans
- 7 cups water
- 1 green bell pepper, chopped
- 1 medium onion, chopped
- 3 celery stalks, chopped
- 3 garlic cloves, chopped
- 3 tablespoons Creole seasoning
- Hot cooked rice
- Garnish: sliced green onions or fresh mint leaves

Directions:

In a 4 quart slow cooker, add all the ingredients; dried red beans, water, bell pepper, onion, celery, garlic and Creole seasoning. Cover and cook on a high setting for 7 hours or until beans become tender. It's as simple as that. Serve with hot, cooked rice and garnish with spring onions or mint.

Veggie-Tastic

Easy-Peasy Slow Cooker Burritos

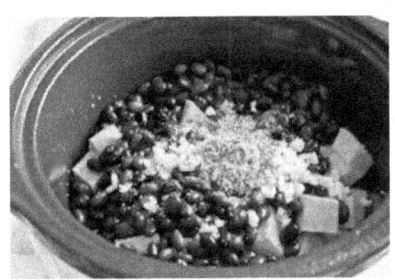

Description: This recipe is extremely simple and requires just a few ingredients but it tastes like something you spent hours working on in the kitchen. The stuffing can even be stored and used to whip up some quick and delicious tacos next time you're in a hurry or have some unexpected guests! Garnish with chopped avocados to add some extra color and flavor.

Ingredients:
- 1 cup brown rice
- 1 teaspoon olive oil
- 2 cups (18 oz.) black bean soup
- 1 cup vegetable broth or water
- Corn tortillas
- Chopped avocados for garnishing

Directions:

Grease the slow cooker with olive oil and add the brown rice, broth and black bean soup. Cook for five hours on a low setting and your stuffing is ready. Scoop into corn tortillas and sprinkle avocado on top.

Vegan Chinese Chow Mein

Description: Who could have thought vegan Chow Mein could taste so good? Carrots, celery and vegan chicken tango with soy sauce and ginger to produce an overpoweringly mouthwatering, slow- cooked Chow Mein.

Ingredients:
- 1 lb. vegan chicken, chopped
- 1 ½ cups celery, chopped
- 1 ½ cups carrots, chopped
- 6 scallions, chopped
- 1 cup vegetable broth
- 1/3 cup soy sauce
- ¼ teaspoonful red pepper flakes
- ½ teaspoonful ginger
- 1 can bean sprouts, drained
- 1 can sliced water chestnuts (8 oz. can)
- ¼ cup cornstarch
- 1/3 cup water
- Noodles or rice for serving

Directions:

Add the vegan chicken, celery, carrots, scallions, broth, soy sauce, pepper flakes, ginger, bean sprouts and water chestnuts to a slow cooker. Put on the lid and cook on a low setting for approximately 7 hours.

Mix the cornstarch and water in a bowl until the texture becomes smooth. Stir the mixture into the crock pot. Cook for two minutes (or until thick) with the lid askew, allowing steam to escape.

Serve with rice or noodles.

Grilled Tofu In Sweet And Sour Sauce With Pineapples

Description: It's easy and it's delicious; what reason could there possibly be for not trying it out? An exquisite balance of flavors and composition, this is a delightful dish that will entice your senses. The sweet, juicy pineapples paired with smoked tofu and seasoned with ginger and soy sauce result in a dish with just the right amount of zest and twang.

Ingredients:
- 1 batch smoked tofu, pressed and cubed
- 2 cups carrot, sliced
- 1 onion, cut in half and sliced thinly
- 2 tablespoonfuls soy sauce, low sodium 2 – 3 tsp fresh ginger, minced or grated
- 1 can pineapple in juice (20 oz. can)
- 3 tablespoonfuls cornstarch
- 3 tablespoonfuls cold water

- 2 cups bell pepper, sliced thinly
- 2 cups broccoli, cubed (or any other vegetable of your choice)

Directions:

Open the can of pineapples and drain the juice into a bowl. Add soy sauce and ginger to the juice to make the sweet and sour sauce. To a slow cooker; add the carrots, sweet and sour sauce and tofu and cook on a low setting for 6 to 8 hours.

In a bowl, mix corn starch and water to make a thickener to be used later.

For the last step; add peppers, broccoli, pineapples and onion to the crock pot and turn the setting on high. Add the thickener to the rest of the ingredients. This last step should usually be performed 45 minutes to an hour, before serving. Let all the ingredients cook until the sauce thickens and the broccoli appears to be done.

Crock Pot Vegan Pot Roast

Description: Golden brown vegetables served with a well-cooked seitan swimming in a delicious, gravy makes this a temptingly satisfying meal for any time of day. Infused with the flavor of thyme and tamari, in every spoonful; this is one pot roast you can't stop eating.

Ingredients:
- 1 box Seitan Quick Mix (6 oz. box)

- ½ teaspoonful onion powder
- ½ teaspoonful dried thyme
- ½ teaspoonful salt
- 1/8 teaspoonful black pepper
- ½ cup water, or more as needed
- 3 tablespoonfuls tamari or other soy sauce
- 1 tablespoonful olive oil
- 2 small sweet yellow onions, halved or quartered
- 1 lb. baby carrots
- 1 lb. small new potatoes, halved or quartered
- Salt and pepper, to taste
- 1 ½ cups vegetable stock
- ¼ cup dry red wine
- 2 garlic cloves, crushed
- 1 teaspoonful thyme

Directions:

Add the seitan mix, onion powder, thyme, salt and pepper to a large bowl and slowly add water while stirring. Also add 2 tablespoons of tamari. Mix the ingredients well; add more water if the mixture appears to be dry. Start kneading the dough, for about three minutes or until it is smooth.

In a large pan, heat oil and add onions, carrots and potatoes. Sauté until golden brown and season with salt and pepper. Add the vegetables and the kneaded dough to a 5 ½ to 6 quart crock pot. Pour in the stock, wine, remaining tamari, garlic and thyme. Cover the cooker and allow ingredients to cook for 7 ½ to 8 hours on a low setting.

Remove the seitan and vegetables from the crock pot and slice the seitan to present it on a serving platter. Surround it with the vegetables and spoon the gravy over it. This recipe makes 4 servings.

Breads, Desserts, And Sweets

Fudgy Peanut Butter Cake

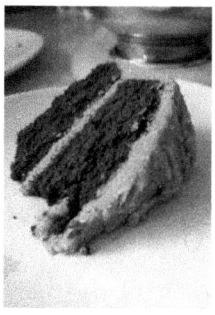

Description: A warm, moist and chocolate-y, peanut butter cake that requires just a few simple ingredients. We know you're going to love it! The heavenly flavor of the warm cake, coupled with some vegan ice cream makes for a delightfully splendid dessert.

Ingredients:
- ½ cup sugar + ¾ cup
- 1 cup flour
- 3 tablespoonfuls cocoa powder + ¼ cup
- 1 ½ teaspoonfuls baking powder

- ½ cup soy milk
- 2 tablespoonfuls nondairy margarine, melted
- 1 teaspoonful vanilla
- 2 cups boiling water
- ½ cup peanut butter

Directions:

Spoon the flour, ½ cup sugar, 3 tablespoons cocoa powder and baking powder into a mixing bowl and stir ingredients to combine. Pour in soy milk, margarine and vanilla and whisk until smooth. Grease a slow cooker and pour in the batter.

Combine boiling water with peanut butter and whisk until texture is smooth. In another bowl, combine the ¾ cup sugar and ¼ cup cocoa. Add the two mixtures together and stir until they are combined well. Pour the mixture over the batter in the slow cooker. Put on the lid and cook for 2 to 2 ½ hours on a high setting or until a toothpick inserted into the center comes out clean.

Serve with vegan ice cream.

Crock Pot Bread Pudding

Description: If you're looking for a bread pudding recipe that balances the proportion of spice with just the right amount of sweetness, you've find yourself a keeper. This simple recipe blends the exotic flavors of cinnamon and nutmeg with crunchy pecans and walnuts to produce a superbly tasty French toast bread pudding.

Ingredients:
- 8 cups soft white Italian bread cubes
- 6 oz. soft or silken tofu, drained
- ½ cup packed light brown sugar
- 2 teaspoonfuls pure vanilla extract
- 1 teaspoonful ground cinnamon
- ¼ teaspoonful ground nutmeg
- 1/8 teaspoonful allspice
- ¼ teaspoonful salt
- 2 cups plain unsweetened non-dairy milk
- ¼ cup pure maple syrup, plus more for serving
- 1 tablespoonfuls non-dairy margarine
- ¼ cup coarsely chopped pecans or walnuts

Directions:

Spread bread cubes on a tray and bake in an oven preheated to 275 degrees Fahrenheit for half an hour. This procedure will allow the bread to dry out.

Blend tofu, sugar, vanilla, cinnamon, nutmeg, allspice and salt in a food processor. Stir in milk and maple syrup.

Spray the inside of a crock pot with cooking spray or grease with oil and transfer the dried bread into it. Pour the milk mixture on top of the cubes pressing with a spoon to moisten the bread. Dot with some margarine and sprinkle pecans or walnuts before putting on the lid and cooking on a high setting for approximately 1 ½ hours. Serve with additional maple syrup.

Heavenly Vegan Chocolate Cake

Description: Looking for a vegan dessert that can be prepared in your slow cooker? Look no further! Moist, spongy and rich; this chocolate cake is exquisitely appetizing and a delightful dessert after every meal. Add some fresh fruits to the side and a sprinkling of icing sugar to change it up or have it just so; this is one sweet treat you would not want to miss out on.

Ingredients:
- 2 ¼ cups flour
- ½ cup unsweetened cocoa powder
- 1 ½ teaspoonful baking soda
- ¾ teaspoonful salt
- 1 ½ cups sugar
- 1 ½ cups hot water
- ½ cup oil (olive or vegetable)
- 1 ½ teaspoonful vanilla
- 1 ½ teaspoonful vinegar

Directions:

Prepare slow cooker by greasing it and turn it on high while mixing the batter.

For the batter, add flour, cocoa powder, baking soda and salt to a large bowl and mix until all the ingredients are well combined. In another bowl add the sugar and hot water and beat with a whisk. Then add oil, vanilla and vinegar. Start spooning in the dry mixture and continue whisking until all the ingredients are well combined and the texture becomes smooth.

Pour the batter into the slow cooker and cook for approximately an hour. After an hour, keep checking on it with a toothpick and cook until the toothpick comes out clean. Allow the cake to cool down before removing from the slow cooker.

Lemon Blueberry Oatmeal Crock Pot Recipe

Description: This recipe combines the tangy zing of lemon with an oomph of blueberries to produce a breakfast that adds a burst of sunshine to your day or gives you the perfect excuse for a dessert. Garnish with finely grated lemon zest and fresh blueberries for that extra flair.

Ingredients:
- ½ cup steel-cut oats
- 2 cups Unsweetened Coconut Milk
- 1 cup blueberries
- 1 teaspoon vanilla extract
- ¼ teaspoon lemon extract (or ½ teaspoon lemon zest)
- 1 – 2 tablespoons sweetener
- For serving: finely grated lemon zest and more fresh blueberries

Directions:

Spray a 1 ½ to 2 quart slow cooker with oil and add oats, coconut milk, blueberries, lemon extract and vanilla extract. Cook on a low setting for 7 to 9 hours (you can cook it overnight). Uncover the crock pot, stir the mixture well to give it a uniform consistency and add the sweetener. Top each serving with fresh blueberries and grated lemon zest.

Apple-Cinnamon Dessert

Description: A straightforward, easy-to-follow recipe that spices up sweet, tender apples with the scent and exquisite flavor of cinnamon. This is a scrumptious addition at the end of any meal!

Ingredients:
- 4 ½cups firm, tart apples, peeled, cored, and sliced
- 2 tablespoonfuls flour
- 1/3 cup white sugar
- 1/3 cup dried cranberries
- ¼ teaspoonful cinnamon
- 2/3 cup oats
- 1 cup water
- 3 tablespoonfuls melted non-dairy margarine
- ¾ cup brown sugar

Directions:

Toss in the apples, flour, white sugar, cranberries, cinnamon and oats into a large mixing bowl and stir well.

Pour water into your crock pot and add the mixture, the melted margarine and the brown sugar. Cover and cook on a low setting for 4 to 5 hours or until apples appear to be tender. This recipe serves 6.

Cream of Asparagus

Preparation Time: 20 minutes
Cooking Time: 4.5 hours
Servings: 4
  Ingredients
1/4 cup margarine
1 onion
3 stalks of celery
3 tablespoons all-purpose flour
4 cups water
1 (10.5 ounce) can condensed vegetable broth
4 tablespoons bouillon powder
1 potato
1 pound fresh asparagus
3/4 cup half-and-half
1 tablespoon soy sauce
1/4 teaspoon ground black pepper
1/4 teaspoon ground white pepper
Directions
1. Peel the potato and dice it thinly.
2. Peel the onion and chop it finely.
3. Chop the celery into small pieces.
4. Trim the excess of the asparagus and dice it thinly.
5. In a slow cooker, melt the margarine and fry the onion for 3 minutes or until they become tender.
6. Throw in the celery and toss for another 3 minutes.

7. Add in the potato, asparagus and toss for about 5 minutes.
8. In a bowl combine the flour with the vegetable broth.
9. Pour that mixture into the slow cooker.
10. Add in the soy sauce, half and half, white pepper, black pepper, and bouillon powder.
11. Give it a good stir and check the seasoning for taste.
12. Cover with lid and cook on low heat for 4 hours.
13. Serve hot with a piece of asparagus on top as a garnish.

Pumpkin, sweet potato and carrot soup

Preparation Time: 30 minutes
Cooking Time: 6 hours
Servings: 6-8
Ingredients
4 carrots
½ of a pumpkin
2 sweet potatoes
1 (10.5 Oz) can cream of mushroom soup
1/3 cup melted butter
Fresh coriander
1 tbsp baking soda
2 onions
5 cups of vegetable broth
1 cup almond milk

Salt and ground black pepper to taste
Directions
1. Dice the carrots into thin cubes.
2. Peel the pumpkin and deseed it.
3. Dice it into thin cubes.
4. Peel the sweet potatoes and chop them into small pieces.
5. Peel the onion and chop them finely.
6. Chop the fresh coriander finely.
7. In a slow cooker melt the butter.
8. Fry the onion for 4 minutes.
9. Add in the sweet potatoes, carrots, pumpkin and toss for about 10 minutes.
10. Add in the baking soda, almond milk, vegetable broth, mushroom soup and give it a good stir.
11. Add the salt and pepper and sprinkle the coriander on top.
12. Cover with lid.
13. Cook on low flame for nearly 6 hours.
14. Once you are happy with the texture, take off the heat and serve hot with bread.

Chickpea Carrot Potato Celery Stew

Preparation Time: 30 minutes
Cooking Time: 6 hours
Servings: 6
Ingredients
1 pound chickpea
4 carrots
2 large red tomatoes

1 tbsp baking soda
2 red onions
6 cups vegetable broth
1/3 cup melted butter
Salt and ground black pepper to taste
Fresh coriander
2 tbsp ginger garlic paste
3 garlic cloves
2 green chilies

Directions
1. Dice the carrots into thin cubes.
2. Cut the red tomatoes into thin slices.
3. Split the green chilies.
4. Mince the garlic cloves.
5. Chop the coriander.
6. In a slow cooker, throw in the chickpeas.
7. Pour the vegetable broth on top of the chickpeas.
8. Cover with lid and cook on low flame for 4 hours.
9. In a pan, melt the almond butter and fry the garlic and onion.
10. Add the carrots, chilies, ginger garlic paste, tomatoes and stir for about 10 minutes.
11. Add the seasoning to it and give it a good stir.
12. Add the mixture to the slow cooker.
13. Add in the baking soda.
14. Stir well and cover with lid again.
15. Cook on medium heat for 2 more hours.
16. Serve hot with tortillas or any bread of your choice.

Creamy Green Bean and Potato Soup

Preparation Time: 20 minutes
Cooking Time: 3 hours
Servings: 4

Ingredients

3 cups fresh green beans
1 (10.5 Oz) can cream of mushroom soup
1 tbsp baking soda
1 1/2 cups peeled and diced potatoes
1/2 cup diced onion
1/3 cup mushroom slices
3 cups almond milk
1/3 cup melted butter
Salt and ground black pepper to taste

Directions

1. Trim the green beans and cut them into 1 inch pieces.
2. In a slow cooker add the green beans and the potatoes.
3. Pour water to cover the green beans.
4. Add baking soda to it and give it a good stir.
5. Cover with lid and turn the heat to low. Cook for 1 hour on low flame.
6. In another pan, melt the almond butter and fry the onions for about 5 minutes.
7. Add the sliced mushroom and toss for about 10 minutes.
8. Now pour the mushroom mixture into the slow cooker. Add the almond milk, mushroom soup to it.

9. Cover with lid and cook on low flame for nearly 2 hours. Serve hot with bread.

Bean Tomato Soup

Preparation Time: 20 minutes
Cooking Time: 2.5 hours
Servings: 4

Ingredients
2 (15 Oz) cans black beans
1 tbsp vegetable oil
1 (8.75 Oz) can whole kernel corn
1 onion, chopped
4 cups vegetable stock
2 carrots
1 tsp ground cumin
1/4 tsp ground black pepper
2 tsp chili powder
1 clove garlic, minced
1 (14.5 Oz) can stewed tomatoes

Directions
1. Rinse and drain the black beans.
2. Chop the carrots into small chunks.
3. In a slow cooker, heat the vegetable oil and fry the garlic, onion, carrots and stir for about 5-8 minutes.
4. Sprinkle the chili powder and cumin in and toss for another 2 minutes.
5. Pour in the rest of the ingredients.
6. Give it a good stir.
7. Take off the heat and pour into a blender.
8. Blend until the mixture is smooth.

9. Transfer the mixture to a slow cooker.
10. Cover with lid and cook on low flame for 2 hours.
11. Serve hot with bread.

Kale and White Bean Soup

Preparation Time: 20 minutes
Cooking Time: 2 hours
Servings: 4

Ingredients

2 tbsp extra-virgin olive oil
1 onion
3/4 cup diced carrot
4 cloves garlic
3 cups low-sodium vegetable broth
2 cups water
1 cup white wine
3 potatoes, halved and sliced
1/2 tsp chopped fresh rosemary
1/2 tsp chopped fresh sage
1/2 tsp chopped fresh thyme
1 (16 Oz) can cannellini beans
2 cups finely chopped kale leaves
1 small red chili pepper
Ground black pepper to taste

Directions

1. Peel and dice the onion. Mince the garlic.
2. Rinse and drain the beans.
3. Deseed the chili pepper and chop it finely.
4. In a slow cooker, heat the oil and fry the onion for about 5 minutes or until it becomes translucent.

5. Add in the garlic and the carrots to the slow cooker.
6. Toss for another 5 minutes. Now pour in the white wine, water, vegetable broth to it.
7. Throw in the potatoes, sage, thyme and rosemary.
8. Give it a good stir and cover with the lid.
9. Turn the heat to medium low and cook for 1 hour.
10. Now add the beans, chili pepper, kale and black pepper to it.
11. Sprinkle in some salt.
12. Again cover with lid and cook on low flame for about 1 hour.
13. Serve hot with crackers or bread.

Vegetable and Lentil Stew

Preparation Time: 20 minutes
Cooking Time: 3 hours
Servings: 4
  Ingredients
1/2 cup red lentils
1 cup chopped onion
1 stalk celery
2 cups shredded cabbage
1 (28 Oz) can whole peeled tomatoes
2 cups vegetable broth
3 carrots
1 clove garlic
1 tsp salt
1/2 tsp ground black pepper
1/4 tsp white sugar

1/2 tsp dried basil
1/2 tsp dried thyme
1/4 tsp curry powder
Directions
1. Mince the garlic and chop the celery.
2. Chop the tomatoes into medium chunks.
3. Chop the carrots finely.
4. Use a slow cooker and add the red lentils.
5. Add enough water to cover the lentils.
6. Cover with lid and cook for 1 hour.
7. Now drain the liquid and again throw the lentils into the slow cooker.
8. Add the celery, onion, tomatoes, carrots, cabbage, and garlic.
9. Pour in the vegetable broth.
10. Give it a good stir.
11. Add in the curry powder, thyme, basil, black pepper and salt.
12. Cover with lid and cook on low flame for about 2 hours.
13. Serve hot with rice or bread.

Stuffed Bell Pepper in Slow Cooker

Preparation Time: 30 minutes
Cooking Time: 4 hours
Servings: 6
  Ingredients
1 pound mushroom
1 cup cooked rice
2 tbsp ketchup

1 tsp Worcestershire sauce
1 tsp ground black pepper
6 green bell peppers
2 tbsp olive oil
1 (14.5 Oz) can fire-roasted diced tomatoes
1/3 cup water

Directions

1. Chop the mushrooms into thin slices.
2. In a slow cooker heat the olive oil.
3. Throw in the mushrooms.
4. Toss for nearly 5 minutes.
5. Add the tomatoes, ketchup, black pepper, salt, rice, and Worcestershire sauce to it.
6. Stir well and cover with lid.
7. Cook for 30 minutes on low flames.
8. Now take off the heat and transfer to a plate.
9. Take the bell peppers and cut out the stem.
10. Cut in a way as if it looks like a basket into which you can fill your filling.
11. Take the mushroom filling and fill the center of each pepper.
12. Now place the bell peppers into the slow cooker carefully.
13. Cover with lid and cook on low flame for about 3 hours.
14. Serve hot with any sauce.

Bean and Pumpkin Stew

Preparation Time: 20 minutes

Cooking Time: 3 hours
Servings: 4

Ingredients

- 1 tbsp olive oil
- 1 red bell pepper
- 1 onion
- 2 cloves of garlic
- 1 tsp ground cumin
- 1 (15 Oz) can pumpkin puree
- 1 (15 Oz) can black beans
- 1 (14 Oz) can whole kernel corn
- 2 cups vegetable broth
- 1 (8 Oz) can tomato sauce
- 1 tsp fresh cilantro leaves
- Salt and pepper to taste
- 1/2 cup heavy cream, whipped (optional)

Directions

1. Peel and chop the onion. Mince the garlic.
2. Chop the bell pepper into thin slices.
3. Drain the corn and the black beans.
4. Chop the cilantro leaves.
5. Now in a slow cooker heat the oil and fry the onion with the bell pepper.
6. Toss for 5 minutes and then add the garlic to it.
7. Add the cumin and toss for another 2 minutes.
8. Add in the corn, tomato sauce, pumpkin puree, vegetable broth, black beans, and the cilantro leaves.
9. Season with salt and pepper.
10. Give it a good stir.

11. Cover with lid and turn the heat to low.
12. Cook for 3 hours.
13. Garnish with the whipped cream on top and serve hot.

Chili Corn Carne

Preparation Time: 20 minutes
Cooking Time: 4 hours
Servings: 4
  Ingredients
1 large onion
1 clove of garlic
2 tsp tomato paste
2 tbsp butter, cut into pieces
2 tbsp olive oil
2 tbsp all-purpose flour
1 tsp dried oregano
1/2 tsp ground cumin
1 1/2 tsp chili powder
1 (14.5 Oz) can whole peeled tomatoes with liquid
1 pound Mushroom
1 (15.25 Oz) can kidney beans
Salt to taste
Pepper to taste
Directions
1. Peel the onion and chop it finely.
2. Mince the garlic and chop the tomatoes.
3. Crush the dried oregano.
4. Chop the mushrooms into thin slices.
5. Rinse and drain the beans.

6. In a slow cooker, heat the olive oil and fry the onion, tomato sauce and the garlic for nearly 10 minutes.
7. Add the almond butter and wait until it melts.
8. Throw in the cumin, oregano, chili powder, mushroom, tomatoes, and flour.
9. Season with salt and pepper.
10. Add enough water to cover the ingredients.
11. Cover with lid and cook on low flame for nearly 4 hours.
12. Serve hot with bread.

Potato and Olive stew

Preparation Time: 20 minutes
Cooking Time: 3 hours
Servings: 4
  Ingredients
2 1/2 pounds potatoes
1/3 cup olive oil
2 cloves garlic
3/4 cup whole, pitted kalamata olives
1 1/3 cups chopped tomatoes
1 tsp dried oregano
Salt and pepper to taste
Directions
1. Peel the potatoes and chop them into small chunks.
2. Mince the garlic cloves.
3. In a slow cooker heat the olive oil and fry the potatoes with the garlic for nearly 10 minutes.
4. Add in the olives, oregano and tomatoes.

5. Season with salt and pepper and pour enough water to cover the potatoes.
6. Give it a good stir.
7. Turn the heat to low and cook for 3 hours.
8. Serve hot.

Hungarian Pea Stew

Preparation Time: 20 minutes
Cooking Time: 4 hours
Servings: 4

Ingredients

3 tbsp vegetable oil
1 onion
2 cloves garlic
3 cups finely shredded Napa cabbage
1 (8 Oz) can sliced water chestnuts
1 pound mushroom
1/8 tsp cayenne pepper
2 bay leaves
1/2 tsp Cajun seasoning
Salt to taste
1 quart vegetable stock
1 (10 Oz) package frozen black-eyed peas
1 1/2 cups basmati rice
3 cups water

Directions

1. Peel and chop the onion. Mince the garlic.
2. Chop the mushrooms into thin slices.
3. Drain the black eyed peas.
4. Rinse the rice well.

5. Drain the water of the chestnuts.
6. In a slow cooker, heat the vegetable oil and fry onion and garlic for 5 minutes.
7. Add in the cabbage, bay leaf, mushrooms, salt, Cajun seasoning and cayenne pepper.
8. Stir for about 10 minutes and pour in the vegetable stock.
9. Cover with lid and cook on low flame for nearly 3 hours.
10. In another pan, add the rice with water and bring the mixture to a boil.
11. Simmer on low flame for 20 minutes. Serve hot with rice on top.

Dal Makhani

Preparation Time: 20 minutes
Cooking Time: 4.5 hours
Servings: 6
  Ingredients
1 cup lentils
1/4 cup dry kidney beans
Water to cover
5 cups water
2 tbsp salt
2 tbsp vegetable oil
1 tbsp cumin seeds
4 cardamom pods
1 cinnamon stick, broken
4 bay leaves

6 whole cloves
1 1/2 tbsp ginger paste
1 1/2 tbsp garlic paste
1/2 tsp ground turmeric
1 pinch cayenne pepper
1 cup canned tomato puree
1 tbsp chili powder
2 tbsp ground coriander
1/4 cup butter
2 tbsp dried fenugreek leaves
1/2 cup cream

Directions
1. Soak the kidney beans and the lentils in water for nearly 2 hours or longer if you can afford the time. Drain well and set aside for now.
2. In a slow cooker throw in the lentils and the kidney beans and pour enough water to cover the beans.
3. Add salt to it and cover with lid.
4. Cook for 1 hour.
5. Now in another pan heat the vegetable oil and fry the cumin seeds, cinnamon stick, cardamom, fenugreek leaves and bay leaf.
6. Throw in the all the pastes, cayenne pepper, coriander, chili powder and turmeric powder.
7. Give it a good stir and add the tomato puree to it.
8. Toss for 6 minutes and then add the mixture to the slow cooker.
9. Cover with lid again and turn the heat to low.
10. Cover with lid again and turn the heat to low.

11. Cook for 4 hours.
12. Add the cream to it and cook for another 30 minutes.
13. Serve hot with rice or bread.

Carrot soup

Preparation Time: 20 minutes
Cooking Time: 3 hours
Servings: 4

Ingredients

3 pounds carrots, chopped
6 cups vegetable stock
3 cloves garlic, chopped
2 tbsp dried dill weed
1/4 pound butter
1 1/2 tsp salt

Directions

1. In a slow cooker pour the vegetable stock, garlic, dill weed, butter, carrots.
2. Add the salt.
3. Give it a good stir.
4. Cover with lid and turn the heat to low.
5. Cook for 3 hours.
6. Serve hot with crackers or chips.

Pumpkin soup

Preparation Time: 20 minutes
Cooking Time: 3 hours
Servings: 4

Ingredients

- 1 2/3 pounds sugar pumpkin
- 2 carrots
- 2 onions
- 2 1/2 tbsp vegetable oil
- 1 large potato
- 1 quart water
- 1 cup heavy cream
- 1 1/4 tbsp ground nutmeg
- 1 tsp ground black pepper
- Salt to taste

Directions

1. Peel the pumpkin and deseed it.
2. Cut it into small chunks.
3. Chop the carrots into thin slices.
4. Peel and chop the onion.
5. Peel and slice the potato into thin pieces.
6. Use a slow cooker and add the vegetable oil and fry the onion for 3 minutes.
7. Add the carrots, potato, pumpkin and toss for 10 minutes.
8. Add the rest of the ingredients.
9. Give it a good stir.
10. Cover with lid and cook on low flame for nearly 3 hours.

11. Serve hot with bread.

Chana Masala

Preparation Time: 20 minutes
Cooking Time: 3 hours
Servings: 4

Ingredients

1 tbsp extra-virgin olive oil
1 small onion
2 cloves garlic
1 (15 Oz) can chickpeas
2 tbsp lemon juice
1 tsp ground coriander
1 tsp ground cumin
1 tsp garam masala
1 tsp curry powder
1/2 cup fresh spinach

Directions

1. Peel the onion and chop it finely.
2. Mince the garlic.
3. Chop the spinach coarsely.
4. In a slow cooker throw in all the ingredients one by one and then add enough water to cover everything.
5. Cover with lid and cook on low flame for about 4 hours.
6. Serve hot with rice or tortillas.

Creamy cauliflower soup with fresh chives

Preparation Time: 20 minutes
Cooking Time: 6.5 hours

Servings: 6

Ingredients

5 tbsp unsalted butter
1 leek
1 onion
1 carrot
1 tsp dried tarragon
1/2 tsp dried thyme
1/4 cup all-purpose flour
1 cup dry white wine
6 cups vegetable stock
Salt to taste
1/4 tsp freshly ground white pepper
1 head cauliflower
1 cup almond milk
1 cup heavy whipping cream
2 1/2 cups shredded Swiss vegan cheese

Directions

1. Peel and chop the onion.
2. Chop the carrots into thin pieces.
3. Separate the cauliflower into small florets.
4. Chop the leek finely.
5. In a slow cooker melt the almond butter and fry the leek, onion, carrots for about 10 minutes.
6. Add all the spices and salt.
7. Add the flour, almond milk, whipping cream, white wine and vegetable stock.
8. Give it a good stir.

9. Cover with lid and cook on low flame for about 6 hours.
10. Add the cheese and cook for another 10 minutes. Serve hot.

Cream of broccoli soup

Preparation Time: 20 minutes
Cooking Time: 4 hours
Servings: 4

Ingredients

1/2 cup butter
1 onion, chopped
1 (16 Oz) package frozen chopped broccoli
4 (14.5 Oz) cans vegetable broth
1 (1 pound) loaf processed vegan cheese food, cubed
2 cups almond milk
1 tbsp garlic powder
2/3 cup cornstarch
1 cup water

Directions

1. In a slow cooker start by melting the butter.
2. Fry the onions golden brown for about 5 minutes.
3. Add in the broccoli and toss for another 5 minutes.
4. Pour in the vegetable broth.
5. Add the garlic powder, almond milk, and salt to it.
6. Give it a good stir and cover with lid.
7. Cook on low flame for nearly 3 hours.
8. Mix the cornstarch with water and pour into the slow cooker.
9. Add the cheese.

10. Cover with lid again and cook for another hour.
11. Serve hot with bread.

Spicy coconut curry soup with broccoli

Preparation Time: 20 minutes
Cooking Time: 3 hours
Servings: 4
  Ingredients
2 tbsp butter
3 leeks
1 clove garlic
1 (32 fluid Oz) container vegetable stock
1 1/2 cups thinly sliced carrots
2 stalks of celery
1 tsp curry powder
1/2 tsp ground turmeric
1/2 tsp ground ginger
1/8 tsp ground black pepper
1 pinch red pepper flakes
1 1/2 (12 Oz) cans light coconut almond milk
Directions
1. Mince the garlic and chop the leeks.
2. Chop the celery into thin slices.
3. In a slow cooker melt the almond butter and fry the leek with the garlic.
4. Toss for 5 minutes or until it becomes golden brown.
5. Add the celery, carrots, ginger, turmeric, curry powder, red pepper flakes, black pepper, almond milk and the vegetable stock.

6. Give it a good stir and ensure that the seasoning is to your desired taste.
7. Cover with lid and cook on low flame for about 3 hours.
8. Garnish with red pepper flakes and serve hot with bread.

Zucchini Soup

Preparation Time: 20 minutes
Cooking Time: 2 hours
Servings: 4

Ingredients

21 Oz zucchini
2 onions
2 cloves garlic
3 cups water, divided
Salt to taste
1 bunch chives

Directions

1. Chop the zucchini into thin slices.
2. Mince the garlic cloves.
3. Peel and chop the onions into thin pieces.
4. Chop the chives into thin slices.
5. Now take a slow cooker and throw in all the ingredients one by one, adding the water at the end.
6. Give it a good stir and check if the seasoning is okay.
7. Cover with the lid and turn the heat to medium low.
8. Cook for 2 hours.
9. Garnish with the chives on top and serve hot with crackers.

Spinach and potato soup

Preparation Time: 20 minutes

Cooking Time: 4 hours

Servings: 4

Ingredients

2 tsp olive oil

4 leeks

2 cloves garlic

2 (16 Oz) cans fat-free vegetable broth

2 (16 Oz) cans cannellini beans

2 bay leaves

2 tsp ground cumin

1/2 cup whole wheat couscous

2 cups packed fresh spinach

Salt and pepper to taste

Directions

1. Chop the garlic and the leeks into thin slices.
2. Rinse and drain the beans.
3. In a slow cooker heat the olive oil and fry the leeks with the garlic for 5 minutes.
4. Add the bay leaves, cumin, beans, spinach, couscous and the vegetable broth to it.
5. Check the seasoning for taste and stir well.
6. Cover with the lid and cook on low flame for about 4 hours.
7. Serve hot.

Thick kidney bean soup

Preparation Time: 20 minutes

Cooking Time: 5 hours
Servings: 4
  Ingredients
1 pound mushroom
3 carrots
3 celery sticks
1 cup canned whole tomatoes
1 onion
2 (19 Oz) cans kidney beans
2 potatoes
Salt to taste
  Directions
1. Chop the carrots into thin pieces.
2. Chop the mushrooms into thin slices.
3. Peel and chop the onion into thin pieces.
4. Peel and dice the potato into small chunks.
5. Rinse and drain the beans.
6. Chop the tomatoes into medium chunks.
7. Now take a slow cooker and add all the ingredients one by one.
8. Pour enough water to cover every ingredient.
9. Cover with a lid and cook on low flame for 5 hours.
10. Serve hot with bread.

Mexican chili con carne

Preparation Time: 20 minutes
Cooking Time: 3 hours
Servings: 4
  Ingredients
2 tomatoes

10 fresh chili de arbol peppers
1 clove garlic
2 tsp vegetable oil
2 pounds mushroom
Salt and pepper to taste
1 cube tomato-flavored bouillon

Directions

1. Chop the arbol peppers.
2. Dice the tomatoes into thin slices.
3. In a slow cooker, heat the vegetable oil.
4. Fry the garlic for about 2 minutes.
5. Throw in the tomatoes, peppers, and the mushroom.
6. Toss for about 10 minutes.
7. Add in the tomato flavored bouillon, and season with salt and pepper.
8. Stir well and cover with lid.
9. Cook on low heat for about 3 hours.
10. Serve with crackers or tortillas.

Kidney beans Carrot Potato Squash soup

Preparation Time: 30 minutes
Cooking Time: 6 hours
Servings: 6

Ingredients

2 tbsp olive oil
1 large butternut squash
1 small yellow onion
1/4 cup finely chopped celery
1/2 cup finely chopped carrot
3 cloves of garlic

2 canned Chipotle peppers in adobo sauce, chopped
1 tbsp chopped fresh basil leaves
1 tbsp chopped fresh parsley
1 tsp cumin
1 (15 Oz) can tomatoes
2 quarts vegetable broth
1 (15.5 Oz) can cannellini beans
1 cup corn kernels
2 limes
1 (10 Oz) bag tortilla chips
1 cup sour cream, for topping
1 (8 Oz) package shredded Mexican blend vegan cheese, for topping

Directions
1. Dice the tomatoes.
2. Cut the limes into wedges.
3. Mince the garlic cloves.
4. Peel the squash and deseed it. Cut it into 1 inch cubes.
5. Peel and chop the yellow onion.
6. In a slow cooker heat the olive oil and fry the squash for 5 minutes or until it gets softened.
7. Throw in the onion, carrots and the celery and toss for another 5 minutes.
8. Add in the basil, garlic, parsley, cumin and chipotle peppers.
9. Throw in the tomatoes and pour in the vegetable broth.
10. Add in the corn kernels, beans.

11. Give it a good stir and check the seasoning.
12. Cover with the lid.
13. Cook on low flame for nearly 6 hours.
14. Garnish with the lime wedges and sour cream on top.
15. Serve hot with bread.

French onion soup

Preparation Time: 20 minutes
Cooking Time: 3 hours
Servings: 4

Ingredients

5 onions
6 cups vegetable broth
2 tbsp vegetable oil
3 tbsp almond butter or margarine
1 pound shredded Swiss vegan cheese
1 tsp white sugar
1/2 cup white wine
Salt and pepper to taste
1 (1 pound) loaf French bread

Directions

1. Peel and chop the onions into thin slices.
2. Slice the loaf of French bread into thin slices and set aside for now.
3. In a slow cooker, heat the vegetable oil and fry the onions for 5 minutes or until it becomes tender.
4. Add the white sugar, white wine, butter, vegetable broth, salt and pepper.
5. Give it a good stir and cook on low flame for 3 hours.

6. Now pour the soup into separate serving bowls.
7. Add one slice of bread on each bowl and top it with the swiss cheese.
8. Place the bowls into the oven and heat until the cheese melts.
9. Serve hot.

Mushroom cream soup

Preparation Time: 20 minutes
Cooking Time: 3 hours
Servings: 4

Ingredients

5 cups sliced fresh mushrooms
1 1/2 cups vegetable broth
1/2 cup chopped onion
1/8 tsp dried thyme
3 tbsp butter
3 tbsp all-purpose flour
1/4 tsp salt
1/4 tsp ground black pepper
1 cup half-and-half
1 tbsp sherry

Directions

1. In a slow cooker throw in the mushrooms, butter, thyme, onion, sherry, all purpose flour, salt and pepper.
2. Add the half-and-half and the vegetable broth to it.
3. Give it a good stir.
4. Cover with the lid and turn the heat to medium low.
5. Cook for 4 hours.

6. Serve hot with bread.

Cream of potato with herbs and green onions

Preparation Time: 20 minutes
Cooking Time: 2 hours
Servings: 4

Ingredients

2 tbsp unsalted butter
1 medium yellow onion
1 1/2 pounds russet potatoes
6 cups water, divided
2 bay leaves
2 large sprigs fresh thyme
8 mushrooms
1 bunch kale
1/4 tsp Salt
1/2 tsp coarsely ground pepper
1 cup whipping cream
1 red apple

Directions

1. Peel and chop the onion.
2. Peel and cut the potatoes into small cubes.
3. Cut the kale into small chunks.
4. Chop the mushrooms into thin slices.
5. Peel the red apple and cut it into thin slices, set aside for now.
6. In a slow cooker melt the almond butter and fry the onion for 5 minutes.
7. Fry the potatoes for 2 minutes and then add enough water to cover the potatoes.

8. Add a pinch of salt, thyme and bay leaf.
9. Cover with lid and cook on low heat for 1 hour.
10. In a pan fry the mushrooms for nearly 10 minutes.
11. Add the mushroom to the slow cooker.
12. Add the kale to it.
13. Check the seasoning.
14. Add the whipped cream to it and cook on low heat for another hour.
15. Garnish with the red apple and serve hot with bread.

Thai mushroom soup

Preparation Time: 20 minutes
Cooking Time: 3 hours
Servings: 4
  Ingredients
1 pound white mushroom
4 cups water
2 lemongrass
4 kaffir lime leaves
4 slices galangal
4 chili padi (bird's eye chili)
1 1/2 tbsp fish sauce
1 1/2 limes, juiced
1 tsp white sugar
1 tsp hot chili paste
1 tbsp tom yum soup paste (optional)
  Directions
1. Take the lemongrass and trim the excess.

2. In a slow cooker throw in all the ingredients one by one.

3. Ensure that the seasoning is to your desired taste and cover with lid.

4. Cook on low heat for nearly 3 hours.

5. Check the texture, if preferred cook for another hour.

6. Serve hot with crackers.

Fresh vegetable soup

Preparation Time: 20 minutes

Cooking Time: 3 hours

Servings: 4

Ingredients

6 cups vegetable broth

1 (16 Oz) package frozen mixed vegetables

1 (14.5 Oz) can diced tomatoes, undrained

2 potatoes

1 large onion

1/2 cup barley

3 cloves garlic

1 tsp dried parsley

1 tsp dried oregano

1/2 tsp dried basil

1/2 tsp salt

1/2 tsp ground black pepper

1 bay leaf

Directions

1. Peel the potatoes and the onion.

2. Chop the onion into thin pieces.

3. Dice the potato into semi small chunks.
4. Mince the garlic cloves.
5. In a slow cooker add all the frozen vegetables.
6. Pour 6 cup of vegetable broth on top.
7. Add the tomatoes to it with the juice.
8. Gradually add the onion, garlic, oregano, potatoes, barley, salt, basil, bay leaf and black pepper.
9. Give it a good stir.
10. Check the seasoning and cover with lid.
11. Cook on low medium flame for nearly 6 hours. Serve hot with parsley on top.

Corn soup

Preparation Time: 20 minutes
Cooking Time: 2 hours
Servings: 4

Ingredients

1 1/4 (16 ounce) packages frozen corn kernels
1/2 cup butter
1/2 cup almond milk
1 tablespoon white sugar
1 (8 ounce) package cream vegan cheese
Salt and pepper to taste

Directions

1. In a slow cooker throw in the cream cheese with the butter.
2. Add in the corn kernels, the almond milk, and white sugar to it.
3. Give it a good stir.
4. Sprinkle the salt and pepper to it.

5. Cover with lid and cook on high heat for 2 hours.
6. Serve hot with bread.

Khichuri

Preparation Time: 20 minutes
Cooking Time: 4 hours
Servings: 6

Ingredients:

4 medium potatoes 1/2 tsp red chili powder 1/2 tsp sugar 1/2 tsp turmeric powder 1 1/4 cup green gram split 250 gm cauliflower florets 6 cup water (approx.)salt to taste 6 green chilies 1 1/4 cup rice 2 tsp cumin powder 1/2 cup peas

For the Seasoning 4 tbsp. Ghee 2 Bay Leaves 3 Red Chilies Whole 4 Green Cardamoms 6 Cloves 2 Cinnamon 1 inch pieces

Directions

1. Peel the potatoes and cut them into small cubes.
2. In a slow cooker throw in the mong daal.
3. Stir continuously to roast them evenly.
4. Meanwhile, cut the cauliflower florets into semi thick pieces.
5. Split the green chilies into half.
6. When they have become toasted nicely, add in the cauliflower florets to it.
7. Add in the cumin powder, turmeric powder and the chili powder to the slow cooker.
8. Toss for 3 minutes and then add the rinsed and drained rice to it.

9. Pour enough water to cover the rice and green grams.
10. Add in the green chilies, vegetables, bay leaves, red chilies, ghee and the masala paste to it.
11. Give it a good stir.
12. Cover with lid and cook on medium low for nearly 4 hours.
13. Serve hot.

Cabbage Cream Soup

Preparation Time: 20 minutes
Cooking Time: 2 hours
Servings: 4
  Ingredients
1 pound mushroom
2 tbsp. olive oil
3 cloves garlic
2 tsp minced fresh ginger root
1 onion
2 cups cubed butternut squash
2 beets
4 red potatoes
4 carrots
1/2 medium head green cabbage
1 tsp hot pepper sauce
2 tsp dried dill weed
2 tsp dried rubbed sage
2 tsp dried thyme leaves
Salt and black pepper to taste

2 quarts vegetable broth

1 (10.75 Oz) can condensed cream of mushroom soup

1/4 cup red wine vinegar

Directions

1. Peel the onion and the potatoes.
2. Chop the mushroom coarsely.
3. Chop the onion into thin slices and cube the potatoes into small cubes.
4. Dice the carrots into medium cubes.
5. Dice the beets into medium cubes.
6. Shred the green cabbage thinly.
7. Mince the garlic finely.
8. In a slow cooker, heat the olive oil and fry the garlic with the onion.
9. Add the mushroom and toss for 5 minutes.
10. Add the ginger, beets, carrots, potatoes, shredded cabbage and butternut squash.
11. Toss for nearly 15 minutes.
12. Add the dill, sauce, salt, sage, pepper and thyme to it. Stir well.
13. Add in the vegetable broth, red wine vinegar and the cream of mushroom soup.
14. Give it a good stir and turn the heat to medium high.
15. Cook for 2 hours.
16. Serve hot with bread or chips.

Slow Cooker Potluck Mushrooms

Preparation Time: 20 minutes

Cooking Time: 5 hours
Servings: 6

Ingredients

2 pound mushroom
1 1/2 cups ketchup
3/4 cup packed brown sugar
1/2 cup vinegar
1/2 cup honey
1/3 cup soy sauce
1 1/2 teaspoons ground ginger
1 teaspoon salt
3/4 teaspoon ground mustard
1/2 teaspoon garlic powder
1/4 teaspoon ground black pepper

Directions

1. Cut the mushrooms into semi thick slices.
2. Take a slow cooker and place the mushroom slices at the bottom.
3. Spread the ketchup on top of the mushroom slices using a spatula.
4. Sprinkle the brown sugar on top.
5. Drizzle the honey, vinegar and soy sauce.
6. Sprinkle the garlic, ginger, mustard, salt and black pepper on top.
7. Turn the heat to high and cover with the lid.
8. Cook for about 5 hours and serve hot.

Easy Slow Cooker Squash

Preparation Time: 20 minutes
Cooking Time: 2.5 hours

Servings: 4

Ingredients

4 pounds yellow summer squash

1 small onion

¼ gm butter

1/4 pound processed vegan cheese food

Directions

1. Cut the processed cheese food into semi thick cubes.
2. Peel the onion and chop it finely.
3. Peel the yellow summer squash and deseed it.
4. Cut the squash into semi thick pieces.
5. Cut the almond butter into cubes.
6. In a slow cooker melt the butter.
7. Fry the onion for 3 minutes or until it becomes tender.
8. Add in the summer squash and cover with lid.
9. Cook on low heat for 2 hours.
10. Add in the cheese and cook for another 20 minutes.
11. Serve hot with bread.

Slow Cooker Tomato Sauce

Preparation Time: 20 minutes

Cooking Time: 10 hours

Servings: 2

Ingredients

10 roma (plum) tomatoes

1/2 small onion

1 teaspoon minced garlic

1/4 cup olive oil

1 teaspoon dried oregano

1 teaspoon dried basil
1 teaspoon ground cayenne pepper
1 teaspoon salt
1 teaspoon ground black pepper
1 pinch cinnamon
   Directions
1. Peel the roma tomatoes. Deseed them. Cut them into slices.
2. Peel the small onion and cut them into thin pieces.
3. In a slow cooker, heat the olive oil.
4. Fry the onion with the minced garlic.
5. Toss for about 5 minutes.
6. Add in the tomatoes and cook for another 5 minutes.
7. Add in the cayenne pepper, basil, cinnamon, oregano, salt and black pepper.
8. Give it a stir and cover with the lid and cook for 10 hours on low flame.
9. Place the contents in a glass jar.

Slow Cooker Jambalaya (Vegan)

Preparation Time: 20 minutes
Cooking Time: 2 hours
Servings: 4
   Ingredients
1 tablespoon olive oil
1 (28 ounce) can diced tomatoes with juice
8 ounces seitan
8 ounces smoked vegan sausage
1/2 large onion
1/2 large green bell pepper

3 stalks celery

1 cup vegetable broth

2 cloves garlic

1 tablespoon miso paste

1 1/2 teaspoons Cajun seasoning

1/2 teaspoon dried thyme

1/2 teaspoon dried oregano

1 cup rice

1 tablespoon chopped fresh parsley

Directions

1. Drizzle the bottom of a 4-quart slow cooker crock with olive oil. Stir tomatoes with juice, seitan, sausage, onion, green bell pepper, celery, vegetable broth, garlic, miso paste, Cajun seasoning, thyme, and oregano into cooker.

2. Cook on low for 4 hours. Add rice to the cooker and cook on High until rice is cooked through, about 30 minutes more. Garnish with parsley.

Breakfast

Slow Cooker Hash Brown Cheesy Potato Breakfast

Preparation Time: 20 minutes

Cooking Time: 6 hours

Servings: 4

Ingredients

Cooking spray

1 (26 ounce) package frozen hash brown potatoes

1 (16 ounce) package bulk vegan sausage

1 (16 ounce) package shredded vegan cheddar cheese
1 cup almond milk
1 tablespoon ground mustard
Salt and ground black pepper to taste

Directions

1. In a slow cooker, spray with the cooking spray.
2. Chop the vegan sausages.
3. Thaw the potatoes.
4. Spread the thawed hash brown potatoes using a spatula or spoon into the slow cooker.
5. In another pan spray with cooking spray and fry the vegan sausages for nearly 5 minutes or until it becomes brown.
6. Stir continuously and make a crumbly mixture.
7. Drain well and get rid of the extra fat or oil.
8. Now throw the crumbly sausages on top of the hash brown potatoes.
9. Use a spatula for spreading.
10. Sprinkle the vegan cheddar cheese on top.
11. Pour the almond milk to it.
12. Add the ground mustard.
13. Season using the salt and ground black pepper.
14. Cover with the lid and cook on low flame for nearly 6 hours.
15. Serve warm.

Apple Breakfast (Easy Slow Cooker Oatmeal)

Preparation Time: 20 minutes
Cooking Time: 2 hours

Servings: 4

Ingredients

4 cups rolled oats

1/2 cup white sugar

1 tablespoon ground cinnamon

1 teaspoon ground nutmeg

1 teaspoon ground ginger

1/2 teaspoon ground allspice

1/4 teaspoon ground cloves

2 1/2 cups water

1 1/2 cups sliced apple

1/2 cup vegetable oil

1 tablespoon molasses

Directions

1. In a slow cooker, throw in the rolled oats.
2. Add the white sugar to it and mix well.
3. Sprinkle the nutmeg, allspice, ground cloves, ground ginger and ground cinnamon to it.
4. Stir well and then add the apple slices, molasses, vegetable oil and 2 cups of water.
5. Give it a good stir.
6. Check the taste and then cover with lid.
7. Turn the heat to low and cook for nearly 5 to nearly 7 hours.
8. Serve warm.

Slow Cooker Fruit, Nuts, and Spice Oatmeal

Preparation Time: 20 minutes

Cooking Time: 10 hours

Servings: 6

Ingredients

2 cups steel cut oats
4 green apples
1 cup dried cranberries
1/2 cup slivered almonds
1/2 cup chopped pecans
3 cups water
1 cup almond milk
1 tablespoon ground cinnamon
1 teaspoon pumpkin pie spice
2 teaspoons butter

Directions

1. Peel the green apples.
2. Get rid of the cord.
3. Cut the apples into thin slices and soak in water until the other ingredients are ready. This would prevent the apple slices from getting blackened.
4. Now take a mixing bowl and throw in the steel cut oats, almonds, cranberries and pecans.
5. Sprinkle the cinnamon and pumpkin pie spice.
6. Add the butter, almond milk and water to it.
7. Give it a good stir.
8. Pour the mixture into a slow cooker.
9. Cover with the lid and cook on low flame for nearly 8 to 10 hours.

Dessert

Slow Cooker Peach Cobbler

Preparation Time: 20 minutes

Cooking Time: 4 hours
Servings: 4

Ingredients

- 3/4 cup old-fashioned oats
- 3/4 cup white sugar
- 2/3 cup brown sugar
- 1/2 cup all-purpose baking mix
- 3/4 teaspoon ground cinnamon
- 5 fresh peaches
- 1 tbsp olive oil or cooking spray

Directions

1. Take a slow cooker and spray with cooking spray or use the olive oil to grease the inside.
2. Peel the peaches and get rid of the pit.
3. Cut the peaches into thin slices.
4. In a mixing bowl combine the white sugar with the brown sugar.
5. Add the all purpose baking mix to it and mix well.
6. Gradually add the oats and the cinnamon and stir well.
7. Finally add in the peach slices.
8. Pour the mixture into your slow cooker and cover with lid.
9. Cook on low flame for 4 hours.
10. Garnish with yogurt and serve cold.

Bread Pudding in the Slow Cooker

Preparation Time: 20 minutes
Cooking Time: 3 hours
Servings: 4

Ingredients

8 cups cubed bread

1 cup raisins (optional)

½ cup of almonds, chopped

2 cups almond milk

2 large bananas

1/4 cup butter, melted

1/4 cup white sugar

1/2 teaspoon vanilla extract

1/4 teaspoon ground nutmeg

Directions

1. Peel and cut the bananas into thin slices.
2. Mash the banana slices and make a smooth paste.
3. Take the bread cubes and place them at the bottom of the slow cooker.
4. Place the raisins on top of the bread cubes.
5. In a large mixing bowl, take the mashed banana.
6. Add the butter, vanilla extract, white sugar, and nutmeg to it.
7. Mix well and then pour the mixture on top of the bread cubes.
8. Cover with lid and cook on low heat for 3 hours.
9. Make sure to do the toothpick or knife check before taking off the heat. If the toothpick or knife check isn't successful, then leave the pudding on the stove for another 30 minutes.
10. Serve cold.

www.ingramcontent.com/pod-product-compliance
Lightning Source LLC
Chambersburg PA
CBHW071438070526
44578CB00001B/137